SLEEP – PHYSIOLOGY, FUNCTIONS, DREAMING AND DISORDERS

NEW RESEARCH ON SLEEP AND SLEEP DISORDERS

SLEEP – PHYSIOLOGY, FUNCTIONS, DREAMING AND DISORDERS

Additional books and e-books in this series can be found on Nova's website under the Series tab.

SLEEP – PHYSIOLOGY, FUNCTIONS, DREAMING AND DISORDERS

NEW RESEARCH ON SLEEP AND SLEEP DISORDERS

OLIVIER RATTÉ
EDITOR

nova
Medicine & Health
New York

NOTICE TO THE READER

Library of Congress Cataloging-in-Publication Data

ISBN: 978-1-53616-882-2

Published by Nova Science Publishers, Inc. † New York

CONTENTS

Preface

New Research on Sleep and Sleep Disorders first addresses how excessive daytime sleepiness is highly prevalent among patients with type 2 diabetes and has been associated with poorer glycemic control. Daytime sleepiness is also associated with cognitive and attention impairment which may lead to sub-optimal self-management and increased medication errors in patients with type 2 diabetes.

Sleep dysfunction has multiple causes in critically ill patients, some of which are extrinsic to the patient and some which are intrinsic to the patient. The disruption of sleep can further destabilize a patient or complicate their ICU course.

In one study, the authors use a network analysis technique to create networks for each of the four "insomnia identity" groups. These findings may help to further understand the role of daytime sleepiness in different insomnia phenotypes and to better target the clinical intervention.

Additionally, the results of a Multiple Sleep Latency Test carried out in forty patients diagnosed with narcolepsy-1 are presented, and protocol is reviewed.

Later, the role of upper cervical spine morphology in the diagnosis and treatment of patients with obstructive sleep apnea is examined. It is suggested that upper cervical spine morphology contributes to phenotypic differentiations between types of obstructive sleep apnea and thereby to its diagnosis, subdivision and treatment.

Some useful knowledge obtained by analyzing the acoustic properties of snoring sounds and the morphological properties of oropharyngeal soft tissues is presented. Snoring sounds and oropharyngeal soft tissues are directly or indirectly related to the severity of sleep apnea syndrome.

Many researchers are moving their attention towards the development of applications for the smartphone related to obstructive sleep apnea syndrome. As such, this compilation analyzes and investigates the functionality of the most accredited apps available for smartphones.

The American Academy of Sleep Medicine and the American Academy of Otolaryngology–Head and Neck Surgery recommend surgery as an option for the treatment of obstructive sleep apnea syndrome, when non-invasive treatments such as CPAP or oral appliances have not been successful. Surgical treatment is more effective when there is an evident anatomical deformity that can be corrected to alleviate the respiratory obstruction.

The concluding study focuses on drugs which induce sleep, such as propofol and dexmedetomidine. Drug-induced sedation endoscopy is a relatively simple way to explore obstruction sites during induced sleep and to give the most precise indication for surgery.

Chapter 1 - Excessive daytime sleepiness is highly prevalent among patients with type 2 diabetes and has been associated with poorer glycemic control. It had been regarded as a major symptom and an indicator of the presence of sleep apnea syndrome (SAS). However, clinical research performed in patients with type 2 diabetes showed that up to 33% of the patients without SAS had excessive daytime sleepiness and excessive daytime sleepiness was absent in up to 22% of those with moderate/severe forms of SAS. Furthermore, Epworth Sleepiness Scale, a sleep apnea screening questionnaire, showed limited sensitivity and specificity failing to identify 15.9% of those type 2 diabetic patients with moderate and severe SAS as being at high risk of SAS. Thus, it has been pointed out that sleep apnea is not the major driver of excessive daytime sleepiness in type 2 diabetes. Other conditions associated with excessive daytime sleepiness in these patients are obesity, sleep deprivation, a lower quality of sleep due to associated co-morbidities, lifestyle and mental and psychological disturbances. Also, it has been shown that another cause of daytime sleepiness in patients with type 2 diabetes is the increased levels of inflammatory cytokines. Currently, cytokines are accepted as mediators of sleepiness and are closely involved in the pathogenesis of type 2 diabetes and its chronic complications. Daytime sleepiness is also associated with cognitive and attention impairment and increased errors which may lead to sub-optimal self-management and increased medication errors in patients with type 2 diabetes which may have an additive effect to cytokines action on the risk of development of diabetes chronic complications.

Chapter 2 - Disruption of sleep in critically ill patients occurs through four mechanisms; decreased total sleep time, alteration of sleep architecture, disturbance of circadian rhythm and fragmentation of sleep. Sleep dysfunction has multiple causes in critically ill patients, some of which arc cxtrinsic to the patient (e.g., a bright and noisy ICU environment), and some which are intrinsic to the patient (e.g., the patient's own underlying illness). Common therapeutic interventions utilized in many critically ill patients, such as common ICU medications and mechanical ventilation, can exacerbate sleep disruption. Disruption of sleep can further destabilize a patient or complicate their ICU course. Simple interventions are important to implement to halt this feedback loop and improve a patient's sleep. Even after recovery, patients are at risk for long-term disruption of healthy sleep due to their prior critical illness.

Chapter 3 - Recently, insomnia has been conceptualized as a continuum or dimensional entity comprising four groups: "complaining poor sleepers [CP]," "noncomplaining poor sleepers [NP]," "complaining good sleepers [CG]," and "noncomplaining good sleepers" [NG]. It is well recognized that sleepiness is one of the daytime impairments in insomnia disorder. However, the importance that daytime sleepiness has in insomnia is not clear-cut. In the last years, sleep researchers have proposed a difference between sleepiness propensity and sleepiness perception. In insomnia, researchers and clinicians suggest that sleepiness perception seems to be more relevant than sleepiness propensity. In this line, a brief sleepiness perception measure, the *Daytime Sleepiness Perception Scale* (DSPS-4), which comprises four items, was developed. In the present study, the authors used network analysis technique to create networks separately for each one of the four "insomnia identity" groups. Data from 673 undergraduate university students were collected. The results showed different network profiles concerning the four sleepiness perception items across the groups. In particular, as to CP group, the most central symptom was item 1 (i.e., During the day, the author feels excessively sleepy, full of sleep) in all the centrality measures considered. These findings may help to further understand the role of daytime sleepiness in different insomnia phenotypes and to better target the clinical intervention to the stronger nodes or symptoms.

Chapter 4 - Multiple Sleep Latency Test (MSLT) is the standard physiological measure of sleepiness.

It conceptualizes sleepiness as the tendency to fall asleep by measuring the speed of falling asleep. Also MSLT has gained acceptance within the field of sleep as standard method of quantifying sleepiness.

In the spring of 1976, Mary Carskadon and colleagues established protocol and development of the MSLT. This test was then formally applied to the clinical evaluation of sleepiness in patients with narcolepsy and later, in patient with OSAS.

The authors present results in MSLT of forty patients diagnosed of narcolepsy-1 and review the actual protocol.

Chapter 5 - The main aim of this chapter is to describe the role of upper cervical spine morphology in diagnosis and treatment of patients with obstructive sleep apnea (OSA).

Pathological conditions of the cervical spine, such as osteoarthritis, cervical osteophytes and osteochondromas, have been reported in relation to OSA. Recently, the morphology of the upper cervical spine in patients with OSA has been described on two-dimensional lateral cephalograms and three-dimensional cone-beam computed tomography. The studies found that the prevalence and pattern of deviations of the upper cervical spine morphology in OSA was different compared to healthy controls. Furthermore, the facial profile including the cranial base was different in

OSA patients with deviations of the upper cervical spine morphology compared to OSA patients without upper spine morphological deviations. In addition, the prevalence and pattern of upper cervical spine morphological deviations in OSA patients seem to affect the outcome of treatment with a mandibular advancement devise (MAD).

Accordingly, it is suggested that upper cervical spine morphology contributes to phenotypic differentiations between types of OSA and thereby to the diagnosis, subdivision and treatment of patients with OSA.

Chapter 6 - As it has been reported that some serious traffic accidents are caused by sleep apnea syndrome (SAS), detection and diagnosis of SAS have increasingly become important in recent years. In this chapter, the authors present some useful knowledge obtained by analyzing the acoustic properties of snoring sounds and the morphological properties of oropharyngeal soft tissues. Snoring sounds and oropharyngeal soft tissues are directly or indirectly related to the severity of SAS. The sections are organized as follows. The first section provides fundamental knowledge regarding snoring sounds and oropharyngeal soft tissues for detection and diagnosis of Obstructive SAS (OSAS) and introduces related studies. The second section describes the differences among acoustic properties of snoring sounds produced by different respiratory routes; oral, nasal, and oronasal inhalation. Since nasal congestion and open mouth during sleep are often regarded as risk factors of OSAS, recognizing such differences is a key to identifying which part is easy to be corrupted when apnea occurs. The third section demonstrates that morphological properties of tongue and soft palate are related to the severity of OSAS. By using the results of the authors' quantitative analysis of MRIs, you can recognize the typical shapes of these soft tissues found in severe OSAS patients. The fourth section focuses on some kinds of unique snores; post-apneic snores. In general, these snores are said to be gasp-like sounds intrinsic to OSAS. But they have not been analyzed in detail, because their nonlinear and nonstationary properties make it difficult to properly calculate the spectra using traditional signal processing techniques. In this section, Hilbert-Huang transform (HHT) designed for analyzing this type of signals is applied to post-apneic snores and their nonlinearity and nonstationarity are quantitatively clarified based on the HHT spectra. Finally, the last section is devoted to a conclusion and future works.

Chapter 7 - Today, the technological aspect of the pathology concerning Sleep Obstructive Disorder Breathing, plays an important role. This is due to the growing response in the global population of this issue and given the significant social and financial costs involved in the diagnostic and therapeutic management. Many researchers are moving their attention towards the development of applications for the smartphone related to OSAS, with different purposes: screening app with scientifically accredited issues such as Epworth Sleepness Scale, Stop Bang, Berlin questionnaire; app to monitor the snoring; app to detect the presence of apnea; apps with therapeutic purposes. For these kinds of applications, the most important requirements of a smartphone are mainly the presence of a high quality sound card with microphone support and a good accelerometer.

The most downloaded apps on the health theme are those about Sleep Disorders Breathing. These apps can be downloaded with google play or Apple store, some are free but others require payment. This work analyzes and investigates the functionality of the most accredited app available on the actual dowloand for smartphone.

Chapter 8 - The American Academy of Sleep Medicine and the American Academy of Otolaryngology–Head and Neck Surgery recommend surgery as an option for the treatment of OSAS, when non-invasive treatments such as CPAP or oral appliances have not been successful or are not tolerated. Surgical treatment is more effective when there is an evident anatomical deformity that can be corrected to alleviate the respiratory obstruction.

According to the American Sleep Apnea Association, a gradual and logical approach must be taken into account when a patient seeks a surgical solution, and it is a fundamental requirement that the patient find a surgeon who understands both the pathophysiology of sleep apnea and anatomy of the upper airways (UA) to guarantee the best chances of success.

The surgical options aim to solve the obstructive problem according to two ways, the first is the reduction of the content, and then acts through the volumetric reduction of soft tissues at the level of UA, most often at the level of palate, uvula, tonsils, adenoids and tongue. The second option aims at enlarging the container, and therefore on more complex interventions to adapt the bony structures of the skull.

Surgical interventions can be schematically divided into nasal surgery, oropharyngeal surgery, hypopharyngeal surgery, laryngeal surgery, multilevel surgery and upper airway by-pass.

The soft palate in the snore-surgery is the anatomical site on which most of the attention has always been concentrated since it is responsible for most of the phenomena of snoring and most of the obstructive ones and has undergone the greatest innovations.

The rationale for palatal surgery is to reduce volume and stiffen a structure that vibrating with the passage of air causes snoring and collapsing causes an obstruction of the UA.

In general, interventions on the palate can be broadly divided into two groups, the first is represented by interventions that have the aim of reduce snoring, and in this case are less invasive surgeries, as the goal is that of stiffening the palate and reducing the excess mucosa that vibrating causes snoring.

The second group consists of interventions that have the aim of reducing above the snoring especially the apnoic episodes, so they are interventions that have a greater invasiveness, since they must stiffen and reconstitute the functionality of a segment of the UA.

In this context, in the last few years great importance has been placed in the surgeon of the oropharynx side wall starting from the Cahali techniques, followed by the Exphansion Sphincter Pharingoplasty by Pang and Woodson up to the innovative techniques such as the Barbed Reposition Pharingoplasty of Vicini and Mantovani.

Chapter 9 - Dynamic airway study during sleep is a clinical challenge in OSAS, in order to target obstruction sites as well as possible. Drug-induced sleep/sedation endoscopy (DISE) was first described by Croft and Pringle in 1991.

According to the "European Position Paper on Drug Induced Sedation Endoscopy (DISE)," written in 2014 by a group of experts of DISE, this exam should be performed in patients affected by disturbing snoring and OSAHS, in whom non-CPAP therapy is considered. DISE may be also be performed in patients who have failed or don't tolerate CPAP therapy.

Moreover, it can be useful to describe why a previous surgery has failed, and how to solve it.

Absolute contraindications to DISE are ASA 4, pregnancy, and patients with an allergy to DISE drugs. Relative contraindications may include morbid obesity.

Talking about drugs to induce sleep, *propofol* and *midazolam* are the most commonly used to perform DISE; *dexmedetomidine* has demonstrated to be suitable as sedative agent too, so it could be used much more in the future.

ENT performing DISE can classify obstruction patterns in several ways, for example with NOHL (Nose, Oropharynx, Hypopharynx and Larynx) or VOTE (Velum, Oropharyngeal wall, Tongue Base, Epiglottis) classifications.

Odontologists can test mandibular advancement devices (MAD) in patients during DISE, in order to set them in the most effective shape to prevent sleep apneas/ hypopneas.

DISE is nowadays a relatively simple way to explore obstruction sites during induced sleep and, finally, to give the most precise indication for surgery (technique and timing); of course it has to be improved in a lot of features: it should be cheaper, quicker, and it should be performed in an almost "natural" sleep.

In: New Research on Sleep …
Editor: Olivier Ratté
ISBN: 978-1-53616-882-2

Chapter 1

Excessive Daytime Sleepiness and Type 2 Diabetes

Adriana Rusu*[*], *MD, PhD
Department of Diabetes and Nutrition Diseases, "Iuliu Hatieganu" University of Medicine and Pharmacy, Cluj-Napoca, Romania

Abstract

Excessive daytime sleepiness is highly prevalent among patients with type 2 diabetes and has been associated with poorer glycemic control. It had been regarded as a major symptom and an indicator of the presence of sleep apnea syndrome (SAS). However, clinical research performed in patients with type 2 diabetes showed that up to 33% of the patients without SAS had excessive daytime sleepiness and excessive daytime sleepiness was absent in up to 22% of those with moderate/severe forms of SAS. Furthermore, Epworth Sleepiness Scale, a sleep apnea screening questionnaire, showed limited sensitivity and specificity failing to identify 15.9% of those type 2 diabetic patients with moderate and severe SAS as being at high risk of SAS. Thus, it has been pointed out that sleep apnea is not the major driver of excessive daytime sleepiness in type 2 diabetes. Other conditions associated with excessive daytime sleepiness

* Corresponding Author's Email: adriana.rusu@umfcluj.ro.

in these patients are obesity, sleep deprivation, a lower quality of sleep due to associated co-morbidities, lifestyle and mental and psychological disturbances. Also, it has been shown that another cause of daytime sleepiness in patients with type 2 diabetes is the increased levels of inflammatory cytokines. Currently, cytokines are accepted as mediators of sleepiness and are closely involved in the pathogenesis of type 2 diabetes and its chronic complications. Daytime sleepiness is also associated with cognitive and attention impairment and increased errors which may lead to sub-optimal self-management and increased medication errors in patients with type 2 diabetes which may have an additive effect to cytokines action on the risk of development of diabetes chronic complications.

Keywords: type 2 diabetes, excessive daytime sleepiness, sleep apnea syndrome, obesity, lifestyle, inflammation

INTRODUCTION

Type 2 diabetes represents the most frequent metabolic disease, with an estimated prevalence in the general population of 3-5% [1]. According to the World Health Organization, 422 million people with diabetes were registered worldwide in 2014. Epidemiologic projections for the year 2045 predict an increase in diabetes prevalence to 693 million [1, 2]. Diabetes` social, economic and medical implications represent a real public health problem. The devastating micro- and macrovascular complications associated with type 2 diabetes lead to increased mortality, 1,5 million deaths due to diabetes being registered worldwide in 2012 [1].

Sleep disruption, either short or long sleep duration, decreased sleep quality or sleep-disordered breathing, has emerged as a modifiable risk factor for type 2 diabetes. Laboratory-based studies in healthy volunteers showed that sleep restriction and changes in sleep architecture are associated with decreased insulin sensitivity [3, 4]. Subsequently, epidemiological studies confirmed the association between sleep disruption and risk of type 2 diabetes independent of the presence of obesity [5].

In humans, metabolism regulation is closely correlated with the sleep-wake cycle [6]. Data from studies on healthy volunteers showed that basal metabolism is reduced by about 15% during sleep, reaching the minimum value during the morning [7, 8]. This decrease in basal metabolism is mainly achieved by glucose metabolism modification consequent to changes in growth hormone and cortisol secretion during sleep. Typically, growth hormone levels are higher when sleeping, reaching peak value during slow wave sleep, while cortisol secretion increases in the second part of sleep, predominantly during REM sleep [9, 10]. These hormonal changes are associated with increased insulin resistance in the first part of sleep, followed by a period of increased glucose utilization and reduced insulin resistance during REM sleep [11]. Thus, any alteration of sleep architecture has potential consequences on carbohydrate metabolism. Also, melatonin shows circadian variation and play an important role in sleep and wakefulness regulation [12]. It also regulates circadian insulin secretion and its dysregulation has been linked to an increased risk for type 2 diabetes [13]. Although the association between sleep disorders and alteration of carbohydrate metabolism has been demonstrated by numerous researches on human subjects and animal models, the mechanisms involved are not yet fully understood.

Excessive daytime sleepiness (EDS) is one of the most frequent sleep disorders in type 2 diabetes. It is defined as the inability to maintain wakefulness during the daytime, especially during low activity or inactivity situations, resulting in sudden sleep onset [14].

This chapter will provide an overview of EDS in persons with type 2 diabetes by summarizing the literature pertaining to sleep disorders in these persons. The pathways linking EDS and type 2 diabetes are described paying attention to metabolic, lifestyle and psychosocial characteristics that may mediate this association and where applicable pointing to a probable bidirectional relationship. Last, but not least the contribution of EDS to deterioration of health status of persons with type 2 diabetes will be outlined.

PREVALENCE OF EXCESSIVE DAYTIME SLEEPINESS IN PATIENTS WITH TYPE 2 DIABETES

Excessive daytime sleepiness is highly prevalent among patients with type 2 diabetes. If in the general population its prevalence is around 12.0% [15], in persons with type 2 diabetes it ranges between 7.2% and 56.7% [16-20]. The difference in reported prevalence in various studies can be explained by the characteristics of patients enrolled. In Asian populations, the prevalence of EDS has been shown to be lower as compared to Latin and Caucasian populations. The largest study performed in Asian populations was the Sankara Nethralaya Diabetic Retinopathy Epidemiology and Molecular Genetic Study (SN-DREAMS) [18] aiming to assess the prevalence of abnormal sleep patterns in persons with type 2 diabetes and their relationship with diabetes chronic complications. This was a population-based cross-sectional study which used a multi-stage sampling technique to ensure representativity of the sample for the Indian population. Of the 1414 participants enrolled, only 7.2% had EDS as assessed by the Epworth Sleepiness Scale (ESS) [18]. Another study performed in five diabetes clinics in India, enrolling 102 persons with type 2 diabetes found a prevalence of EDS of 17.5% [16]. In three studies, two enrolling Caucasian populations with type 2 diabetes and one an African population the estimated EDS prevalence was around 22.0% [17, 20, 21]. The highest prevalence (56.8%) has been reported in a study enrolling 290 Latino persons with type 2 diabetes from Ecuador [19].

ASSESSMENT OF EXCESSIVE DAYTIME SLEEPINESS

The most frequent tool used for the assessment of EDS is the ESS, an easy to use and self-administered questionnaire comprising 8 items that measure subjects' likelihood of dozing off in eight real-life situations [22]. Responses to all items are scored: 0= never doze, 1=low chance of dozing, 2=moderate chance of dozing, 3=high chance of dozing. Total scores range between 0 and 24 and are obtained by summing the responses to individual items. A total score of 11 or more is considered indicative of daytime sleepiness [22]. Of note, ESS evaluates the subjective daytime sleepiness.

Objective evaluation of daytime sleepiness is performed with Maintenance of Wakefulness Test and Multiple Sleep Latency Test. Maintenance of Wakefulness Test is a polysomnographic technique which evaluates the ability to maintain wakefulness during soporific situations, isolated from factors influencing the pressure to fall asleep (ambient temperature, light, noise) [23]. The patient is required to sit in bed in dim light and to stay awake in 4 trials of 40 minutes at 2 hours intervals [24]. Multiple Sleep Latency Test is also a polysomnographic procedure that measures the physiological sleep tendency in a controlled ambient [25]. The test starts 1.5-3 hours post nocturnal sleep, the patient is offered 5 nap opportunities at 2 hours intervals and the time from lights off until sleep onset is recorded [24].

Pathophysiology of Excessive Daytime Sleepiness in Type 2 Diabetes

As illustrated in Figure 1 the pathophysiology of EDS in type 2 diabetes is multifactorial. Among the factors identified, and which are discussed below is the co-existence of sleep apnea syndrome (SAS), short

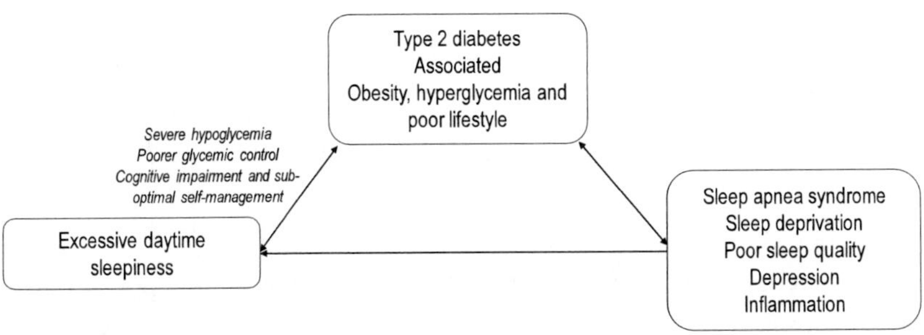

Figure 1. The pathophysiology of excessive daytime sleepiness in type 2 diabetes.

sleep duration, poor sleep quality, and sleep fragmentation, associated systemic diseases, psychological/psychiatric conditions, metabolic changes, lifestyle or adverse effects of medications.

Sleep Apnea Syndrome

Sleep apnea syndrome (SAS) is a sleep-disordered breathing characterized by repetitive episodes of apnea and hypopnea during sleep associated with oxygen desaturation [26]. In persons with type 2 diabetes, its prevalence is significantly higher as compared to the general population, reaching figures ranging between 20.0% and 86.6% of the adults [27-32].

EDS had been regarded as a major symptom and an indicator of the presence of SAS. It is the major complaint of patients addressing for sleep evaluation. In the early stages of SAS research, it was postulated that sleep fragmentation due to SAS is a major determinant of EDS seen in these patients [33]. Subsequent studies showed that SAS patients with EDS had longer sleep duration than those without EDS. Several small studies performed in persons with obesity showed that patients with EDS had higher sleep efficiency and longer sleep duration during the night as compared to those without EDS [34, 35]. Also, subjective EDS was not correlated with polysomnographic measurements in the previous night, and thus it was not a consequence of low sleep quality or short sleep duration in the previous night [34, 35]. These small-scale observations were further confirmed in a large multicenter study in which were enrolled 2882 consecutive patients with SAS from Spain. This study showed that patients with EDS had a longer sleep time, a shorter sleep latency, higher sleep efficiency and deeper sleep depicted by a longer NREM sleep in stages 3 and 4 (11% vs. 8%, $p=0.018$) [36]. Based on these results the authors concluded that neither SAS nor SAS-related sleep disruption is the primary determinants of EDS in these patients [36]. Given that persons with obesity have a higher grade of daytime sleepiness as compared to those without obesity, it has been hypothesized that metabolic changes could explain the sleepiness [33]. Type 2 diabetes is frequently associated with obesity, and obesity has been identified as the main risk factor for SAS in persons with and without diabetes [37]. Thus, obesity-related metabolic changes and not SAS could be the main determinants of daytime sleepiness in persons with type 2 diabetes and SAS.

Furthermore, the association of SAS with EDS is weak both in patients with type 2 diabetes and in general population [34, 38-40]. Our research performed in persons with type 2 diabetes showed that up to 33% of the patients without SAS or with a mild form of SAS had EDS and EDS was absent in up to 22% of those with moderate/severe forms of SAS. Large clinical studies supporting a weak correlation between daytime sleepiness and SAS are also available from the general population. In Pen State Cohort study EDS was reported by only 17% of those with moderate/severe SAS [41, 42], in Wisconsin Sleep Cohort study by only 22% of women and 17% of men with sleep-disordered breathing [43]. Furthermore, the ESS score, the screening questionnaire most frequently used for the assessment of EDS, showed a weak correlation with SAS parameters. In a study enrolling persons with type 2 diabetes, we showed that correlation coefficients of ESS with SAS parameters ranged between -0.29 ($p=0.01$) for mean O_2 saturation and 0.36 ($p=0.002$) for apnea-hypopnea index [44]. In the same study, the sensitivity and specificity were limited (84.1% and 74.1%, respectively) failing to identify 15.9% of patients with moderate and severe SAS as being at high risk of SAS [44]. Additionally, the therapy of SAS with continuous positive airway pressure (CPAP) and correction of apnea-hypopnea index does not lead to remission of EDS in all patients [45]. Rates of residual daytime sleepiness vary between 12% and 30% in patients using CPAP >4 h/night [45, 46]. Also, up to 20% of the obese patients using CPAP ≥7 hours/night have objective sleepiness as assessed by the maintenance of wakefulness test and 20% still present subjective daytime sleepiness as assessed by ESS [46]. These observations further support the idea that SAS is not the major driver of EDS in type 2 diabetes.

Sleep Deprivation and Sleep Quality in Type 2 Diabetes

The frequency of sleep disorders is higher in persons with type 2 diabetes as compared to controls and both short sleep duration and poor sleep quality have been associated with EDS [47, 48]. A meta-analysis assessing sleep duration and patterns in Asian populations with type 2 diabetes, in which were included 47 studies and 98911 patients, showed that the frequency of sleep deprivation (<7 hours/night) was 37.4% in the diabetes group and 14.1% in the control group [49]. Similarly, in a multi-ethnic population comprising in majority Caucasian, Hispanic and Black-Americans with type 2 diabetes the frequency of short sleep duration (<6 hours/night) was 31.9% [50]. The frequency of poor sleep quality is also high in persons with type 2 diabetes, ranging between 34.8% and 81%, depending on the population assessed [51, 52]. In Asian populations, in a small-scale study (46 persons with type 2 diabetes) and using a cut-off of 5 for the Pittsburgh Sleep Quality Index, Tsai et al. [51] reported a frequency of poor sleep quality of 34.8%. Another study, which enrolled 250 Turkish persons with type 2 diabetes reported a prevalence of poor sleep quality of 63.3% [47]. The highest frequency of poor sleep quality (of 81%) was reported in a study enrolling 1211 persons with type 2 diabetes from Jordan [52]. Gender seems to influence sleep quality, with female gender being associated with 2-3 folds higher risk of poor sleep quality [52-54].

Multiple factors have been incriminated as risk factors for sleep deprivation and poor sleep quality in type 2 diabetes: peripheral neuropathy-associated pain, nocturnal hypoglycemia or hyperglycemia, nocturia, associated psychological factors, and comorbidities. Also, it has been shown that diabetes may associate central nervous system dysfunction with neurotransmitter, neuroendocrine and autonomic function alterations which may themselves cause sleep disturbances [55, 56].

Obesity

Obesity is a frequent association of type 2 diabetes and the main risk factor for its development. The prevalence of EDS is high among persons with obesity and several studies have shown that EDS is associated with obesity independent of SAS [34, 35, 57]. In a study comparing the prevalence of EDS in obese vs normal weight persons, Mokhber et al. [58] showed that those with obesity (body mass index [BMI] $\geq$30 kg/m^2) had 2.5 folds higher risk of having EDS as compared to those without obesity (BMI 19.5 - 24.9 kg/ m^2; odds ratio [OR] = 2.493 [95% confidence interval [CI] 1.144 - 5.435]). In an analysis of the Penn State Adult Cohort was showed that obesity at baseline was an independent predictor of incident EDS being associated with 1.8 folds higher risk for the development of EDS during the follow-up (AOR = 1.8, 95% CI = 1.2–2.8, P = 0.011). Also, a weight gain during the follow-up of 2 kg/m^2 or more was associated with 2.8 higher risk of incident EDS (OR = 2.8, 95% CI = 1.8–4.3, P = 0.00006). In this analysis of Penn State Adult Cohort were included 1,395 adults followed for 7.5 years and for which was available at baseline a laboratory sleep study [59]. Similar results were reported from the Sleep and HEalth in women ("SHE") cohort, in which were enrolled 4,322 women without EDS and were followed for 10 years. One of the independent predictors for the development of EDS during the follow-up was the presence of obesity at baseline (OR 1.91; 1.14–2.57) [60]. In the Sleep Heart Health Study during the 5 years of follow-up was observed that every 10 kg increase in the body weight was associated with 0.36 units worsening of the ESS score, and only 17.8% of the relationship between obesity and EDS could be explained by SAS [61]. Vgontzas et al. [34] evaluated the EDS in obese vs. control patients without SAS or other sleep-related pathologies, as confirmed by polysomnography, and showed that obese participants were sleepier than controls. Also, these participants had shorter sleep latencies during a modified sleep latency test, a greater percentage of time spent asleep during the day, a lower percentage of sleep time during the night and a higher percentage of time awake during the night [34]. Sleep time during the night, both short and long sleep duration, have been associated with obesity. Thus, one may think that apart from being involved in the pathogenesis of obesity, short sleep duration may represent the cause of EDS observed in those with obesity without SAS. In the study of Vgontzas et al. [34], nocturnal sleep time was 45 minutes shorter in those with obesity as compared to controls. It is still unclear if this reduction in sleep during nighttime is long enough to result in EDS [62].

Clinical studies showing the improvement of ESS with bodyweight reduction further support the association of obesity with daytime sleepiness. In a study enrolling 158 patients with T2DM and a BMI ≥30 kg/m^2 who were administered liraglutide therapy for at least 3 months, EDS improved (from an ESS score of 6.3 at baseline to 4.2 at month 3) in parallel with bodyweight reduction (from a BMI of 39.6 kg/m^2 at baseline to 37.9 kg/m^2 at month 3). No significant change in body fat was observed after liraglutide therapy suggesting that EDS reduction was independent of changes in body fat. In the same prospective analysis of the Penn State Adult Cohort, Fernandez-Mendoza et al. [59] showed that a weight loss of 2 kg/m^2 during the 7.5 years of follow-up was associated with a 2.5 higher chances for EDS remission (OR = 2.7, 95% CI = 1.4–5.2, p=0.003). Also, a significant improvement in EDS was reported in patients with obesity who underwent bariatric surgery. In a study enrolling 56 obese patients with SAS which underwent gastric bypass, ESS score decreased from 14 before surgery to 5 at 1 month following the surgical intervention [63]. Similarly, Dixon et al. [39] reported a significant improvement of ESS score (from 13 to 3.8) in patients with a mean BMI of 53 kg/m^2 who underwent laparoscopic gastric banding. A meta-analysis including 42 studies evaluating the effect of surgical and non-surgical weight loss interventions on EDS showed an L-shape, non-linear association between weight loss and EDS changes, with a clear dose-response relationship [64]. The amplitude of the effect varied according to the intervention. Clinical studies which evaluated the effect of surgical weight loss on EDS showed a moderate to large effect size of 4.8 points reduction in ESS score [64]. For non-surgical weight loss studies, the effect was small to moderate, an equivalent of 2.6 points reduction in ESS score [64].

Current evidence suggests that EDS is not a precursor of obesity but rather weight gain is an independent predictor of EDS development and thus, that EDS is probably a consequence of metabolic changes occurring in obesity [59, 65]. The mechanisms by which obesity induces EDS are not yet fully understood, but the overactivation of sympathetic nervous system, inflammatory, hormonal and metabolic factors, the development of SAS, and the association with other medical conditions that influence sleep – i.e., type 2 diabetes and depression were suggested [62, 66]. Also, leptin and ghrelin, two of the most important adipokines involved in obesity development, are known to influence metabolism by acting at central nervous system levels and influencing sleep/wake cycle [62]. Leptin levels are known to be high in obesity but also leptin resistance has been described. In animal models, the administration of high leptin doses increased slow sleep [67]. Also, leptin resistance seen in obesity reduces at the hypothalamic level the transcription of cocaine- and amphetamine-regulated transcript (CART), an anorexigenic peptide that promotes wakefulness [68].

Inflammation

Insulin resistance, the main pathogenetic mechanism of type 2 diabetes, has been associated with increased levels of proinflammatory cytokines, such as interleukin (IL)-6, tumor necrosis factor (TNF)-α and C-reactive protein [69]. Inflammation is an important mechanism involved in the association of type 2 diabetes and EDS [70]. Inflammatory cytokines TNF-α, IL-1, and IL-6 have been shown to influence sleep duration. Their levels follow a circadian rhythm with a normal peak during slow-wave sleep, supporting a link between these biomarkers and sleep [71-73]. In patients with EDS, the normal peak of the inflammatory cytokine does not occur during the night, but increased levels have been observed between 6:00 and 7:00 in the morning. Also, patients with EDS display 2 to 3- fold higher levels of these cytokines suggesting their pathophysiological role in the development of EDS [74] and TNF-α, IL-1 and IL-6 administration in humans has been associated with sleepiness and increased sleep duration while the administration of TNF-α antagonist in persons with obesity and SAS improved EDS [75-78]. In a pilot interventional placebo-controlled study in which 8 patients with obesity and SAS received etanercept, a TNF-α antagonist that obstruct its interaction with cell surface receptors, a significant decrease in objective sleepiness, as assessed by multiple latency test, was observed after 3 weeks of therapy in the etanercept group (3.1 ± 1.0 min, $p < 0.05$). Although TNF-α did not change after therapy, a significant decrease in IL-6 levels was observed [75].

Sleep disturbances associated with EDS have been linked to increased levels of inflammatory cytokines independent of obesity, which on the long term has a detrimental effect on glucose metabolism [70, 74, 79]. Chronic increase of these cytokines induces insulin resistance in skeletal muscles [80]. Of these cytokines, IL-6 and TNF-a may alter insulin signaling pathway [81]. Also, elevated FFA levels, frequently associated with insulin resistance due to impaired insulin function, activate toll-like receptors (TLRs) and cytokine response and further alter insulin signaling pathway by activation of Jun N-terminal kinase (JNK) and consequent impairment of tyrosine kinase phosphorylation of serine in insulin receptor substrate-1 (IRS-1) [82]. Resulting insulin resistance and hyperglycemia induce IL-6 production, thus creating a vicious cycle where inflammation induce insulin resistance and hyperglycemia that in turn promote inflammation [83].

Role of Hyperglycemia

Several clinical studies showed that type 2 diabetes is associated with EDS independent of obesity or other risk factors for sleepiness. It has been shown that acute glucose fluctuations may play a role in the EDS seen in diabetes. In a case-control study enrolling 413 persons with type 2 diabetes and 413 controls matched for age, gender, BMI, waist and neck circumference, Lecube et al. [17] showed that ESS score was significantly higher in those with a fasting plasma glucose of 235.8 mg/dl or higher

(ESS=8.6) as compared to those with a fasting plasma glucose below 235.8 mg/dl (ESS=7.1, p=0.005). Also, in the regression analysis fasting plasma glucose was associated with ESS score, independent of polysomnographic parameters [17].

The mechanism likely involved in this association is the effect of hyperglycemia on the orexin neuronal signaling. Orexin is a member of the incretin family and a neuropeptide with pleiotropic effects [84]. Orexigenic neurons are located in lateral hypothalamus and play a role in wakefulness, feeding and glucose regulation [85]. Orexin is an excitatory neurotransmitter involved in promoting wakefulness in response to food deprivation and is released in response to hypoglycemia associated with food deprivation [86, 87]. Low levels of orexin promote sleep and very low levels have been described in coma [88, 89]. High extracellular glucose concentrations inhibit orexigenic neurons and orexin release [90]. Synergistically, in the presence of hyperglycemia, melanin-concentrating hormone (MCH) neurons which promote sleep increase their activity and MCH release [91]. These observations support the hypothesis that hyperglycemia influence daytime sleepiness through its effect on orexin and MCH neuronal activity [62, 92]. In support of these observations are researches in animal models and humans that showed that GLP-1 agonists excite orexin neurons and improve daytime sleepiness [93, 94].

Psychological Aspects of Type 2 Diabetes and Association with Sleep

Type 2 diabetes is frequently related to poor quality of life and psychological disturbance. The prevalence of depression in persons with type 2 diabetes is up to 2 times higher as compared to the general population [95]. Depression is associated with decreased quality of life [96], increased non-compliance with medical recommendations [97] and increased mortality [98]. One of the symptoms of depression is hypersomnia lasting for at least 2 weeks [99]. Thus, EDS in persons with type 2 diabetes may be an expression of depression in these patients and a large body of evidence has shown that depression is an independent predictor of EDS. In the Pen State Cohort comprising a large sample of 16,583 persons from Pennsylvania with age between 20 and 100 years old showed that depression was the most important risk factor for EDS, followed by BMI, diabetes, and SAS [100]. The risk of EDS was 6.8 times higher in those with depression than in those without (OR=6.85, $p < 0.001$) [100]. Zakynthinos et al. [101] assessed determinants of subjective EDS in 915 persons and showed that depression and diabetes were responsible for 11% and 6% of the ESS score variability. In another cohort of participants with obesity, Dixon et al. [102] showed that high Beck Depression Inventory scores were predictors of high ESS score and thus EDS (β=0.15, $p < 0.001$). In a study enrolling 110 persons with type 2 diabetes, Medeiros et al. showed that EDS was associated with the presence of depressive symptoms independent of age, gender, body mass index and glycated hemoglobin (OR=2.27; 95%CI=1.03-5.03) [103].

Lifestyle

In recent years, evidence has accumulated on the effects of lifestyle components – i.e., physical activity and food ingestion – on sleep.

Recent research showed that food restriction promotes wakefulness. Jacobs and McGinty described in animal models that food deprivation progressively increase wakefulness and decrease sleep, an effect that was observable after 4-5 days of complete food deprivation [104]. In another study, also in animal models, it was reported that the weight loss consequent to food deprivation was followed by an increase in wake time [105]. In humans, arousal is an important mechanism for protecting against life-threatening hypoglycemia, particularly in persons with type 2 diabetes treated with hypoglycemiants [106]. Conversely, food intake has been linked to sleep onset. In animal models "cafeteria diet" (a diet high in fat and calories) was associated with increased sleep and decreased wakefulness, which maintained for 3 days after withdrawn of this diet [107]. Several studies enrolling small groups of human volunteers showed that regular intake of fat-rich meals and excess of nutrients are associated with increased subjective and objective day time sleepiness [108-111]. Also, Harnish et al. [108] investigated the effect of ingesting a solid meal versus chewing but not ingesting the meal on objective sleepiness and reported a decrease in sleep latency by 2 minutes in those ingesting the meal. Orr et al. [112] assessed the effect of a solid meal versus water ingestion and of high-fat, high-carbohydrate, or mixed meal on postprandial objective sleepiness and reported a decreased sleep latency in those consuming the solid meal and no difference between meal composition. Wells et al. [113] showed that high-fat low-carbohydrate meals induced sleepiness and sleepiness increased in parallel with cholecystokinin levels. In a rat model, Hansen et al. [114] showed that food-induced sleepiness is associated with changes in IL-1B mRNA in the brain and that cafeteria diet-induced sleepiness can be prevented by vagotomy [115]. Thus, it was hypothesized that sleepiness could be due to hormonal and inflammatory changes induced by high-fat meal (increase in inflammatory cytokines and leptin levels and decrease in orexin, norepinephrine, and serotonin). This hypothesis was further confirmed by a recent cohort study performed in real-life settings. Lopes et al. [116] investigated the effect of the dietary inflammatory index on sleepiness in patients with SAS and showed that patients in the 4th quintile of pro-inflammatory diet (more pro-inflammatory diet) displayed higher ESS scores and more EDS than those with a more anti-inflammatory diet ($p <0.05$). Also, the administration of an IL-1 receptor antagonist (anakinra) in lean and obese subjects decrease subjective sleepiness induced by a high-fat meal [117].

Physical activity is another lifestyle component that has been associated with daytime sleepiness. In a prospective cohort study in which were enrolled 145 persons with type 2 diabetes followed for 2 years, Vasconcelos et al. [118] showed that lower levels of physical activity were associated with EDS independent of age, gender, cardiovascular diseases, waist circumference, and Charlson Comorbidity Index (OR=0.52, 95% CI=0.29-0.92, p=0.02). In a meta-analysis that included 5 studies and 129 participants with SAS, it was shown that exercise training significantly improved EDS (a decrease of 3.3 points on ESS [95% CI -5.57 to -1.02; p=0.004]) independent of changes in body weight [119]. The link between physical activity and EDS is bidirectional, the presence of sleepiness is a risk factor for physical inactivity [120]. Despite proven beneficial effects on glycemic control and quality of life, persons with type 2 diabetes are more likely to be sedentary as compared to the general population. Among barriers incriminated in adopting a more active lifestyle are fatigue usually attributed to high glucose levels, fear of hypoglycemia and micro-and macrovascular chronic complications [121-123].

Hazards of Excessive Daytime Sleepiness in Patients with Type 2 Diabetes

Several consequences of EDS have been identified in persons with type 2 diabetes, such as an increased risk of severe hypoglycemia, poorer glycemic control, cognitive and attention impairment.

A previous study has shown that the presence of EDS is a risk factor for severe hypoglycemia - the Edinburgh Type 2 Diabetes Study, in which were analyzed 898 participants aged 60-75 years of age, recruited between 2006 and 2007, who completed the ESS and for which the history of severe hypoglycemia was available [124]. The study showed that persons with EDS had a higher frequency of nocturnal severe hypoglycemia (15.6% vs. 9.0%, p=0.016). This was confirmed in the regression analysis which showed that EDS was an independent predictor of severe hypoglycemia (Wald statistic=4.939, p=0.026) [124]. Surprisingly, the Berlin questionnaire which assesses the risk of the presence of sleep-disordered breathing was not associated with the risk of hypoglycemia, suggesting that sleepiness as a symptom and not sleep-disordered breathing are risk factors for hypoglycemia. Also, participants with EDS with severe hypoglycemia had higher HbA1c values [124], suggesting suboptimal diabetes management which is a known risk factor for hypoglycemia [125]. In persons with diabetes, severe hypoglycemia is a risk factor for cognitive impairment, cardiovascular events and increased mortality [126-128]. In Edinburgh Type 2 Diabetes Study ≥ 1 episode of severe hypoglycemia was associated with lower cognitive ability in elderly as shown by poorer performance at Letter-Number Sequencing (8.9 vs. 9.8, $p=0.001$), Verbal Fluency (33.8 vs. 37.4, $p=0.006$), Trail Making ($p<0.001$) and Digit Symbol (45.1 vs. 50.0, $p=0.001$) testing, independent of age and gender [126]. By analyzing Medicare data from 860,845 patients, Johnston et al. [127] showed that hypoglycemia is associated with 79% higher odds of acute cardiovascular events than those without hypoglycemia (OR 1.79; 95%CI: 1.69-1.89), independent of age, gender, the presence of chronic kidney disease, peripheral vascular disease, and diabetes chronic complications. Also, severe hypoglycemia is associated with a higher risk of all-cause mortality, 19.9 higher during the first month following the event, as described by Lo et al. [128].

As shown in the Edinburgh Type 2 Diabetes Study, EDS is associated not only with a higher risk of severe hypoglycemia but also with a poorer glycemic control [124]. In a previous study enrolling 242 consecutive persons with type 2 diabetes and obesity, we showed that those with subjective daytime sleepiness had a poorer glycemic control, as assessed by HbA1c (HbA1c 8.5% in those with EDS and 7.3% in those without EDS, $p<0.001$) [20]. The presence of a poorer glycemic control was confirmed in another cross-sectional study performed in India. By analyzing data from this study, Raj et al. [16] showed that HbA1c increased with 14.3% for every unit increase in ESS score ($p<0.001$). More recently, in a larger study including 585 persons with type 2 diabetes, Keskin et al. [129] showed that a significantly lower number of persons with EDS achieve a good glycemic control, defined as an HbA1c $<6.5\%$) as compared with those without daytime sleepiness (34.7% vs. 65.29%, $p<0.001$).

Increased risk of hypoglycemia and poorer glycemic control could be due to sub-optimal self-management of diabetes in these patients. It has been shown that daytime sleepiness is also associated with cognitive and attention impairment and increased errors and these may lead to sub-optimal self-management and increased medication errors in persons with type 2 diabetes which may have an additive effect to cytokines action on the risk of development of diabetes chronic complications [130]. In a study enrolling 107 adults with type 2 diabetes and daytime sleepiness, Chasens et al. [131] showed that daily disturbance factor of the Pittsburgh Sleep Quality Index, which also includes sleepiness, was negatively associated with Diabetes Care Profile, an instrument that assesses psychosocial factors related to diabetes management, including diet and self-care adherence.

Conclusion

The association between EDS and type 2 diabetes is important, because a bidirectional relationship may exist between them. Type 2 diabetes may trigger EDS through multiple mechanisms and in turn, EDS may further impair diabetes control increasing the risk of diabetes chronic complications, cardiovascular diseases, and all-cause mortality. All healthcare providers involved in the care of persons with type 2 diabetes should be aware of what daytime sleepiness is and its implications as outcomes of these patients can be improved by correct evaluation, diagnosis and possible therapy of disorders behind EDS.

References

[1] World Health Organization. 2016. *Global report on diabetes*. Geneva: WHO Press. https://apps.who.int/iris/bitstream/handle/10665/204871/9789241565257_eng.pdf;jsessionid=EB0D425C4A490833C0567112D473B4DF?sequence=1.

[2] International Diabetes Federation. 2017. *IDF Diabetes Atlas*. Eighth edition 2017. www.diabetesatlas.org.

[3] Spiegel, Karine, Leproult, Rachel, and Eve Van Cauter. 1999. "Impact of sleep debt on metabolic and endocrine function." *Lancet* 354:1435–9. doi: 10.1016/S0140-6736(99)01376-8.

[4] Broussard, Josiane L., Ehrmann, David A., Van Cauter, Eve, Tasali, Esra, and Matthew J. Brady. 2012. "Impaired insulin signaling in human adipocytes after experimental sleep restriction: a randomized, crossover study." *Annals of Internal Medicine* 157:549–57. doi: 10.7326/0003-4819-157-8-201210160-00005.

[5] Cappuccio, Francesco P., D'Elia, Lanfranco, Strazzullo, Pasquale, and Michelle A. Miller. 2010. "Quantity and quality of sleep and incidence of type 2 diabetes: a systematic review and meta-analysis." *Diabetes Care* 33:414–20. doi: 10.2337/dc09-1124.

[6] Kovac, Judit, Husse, Jana, and Henrik Oster. 2009. "A time to fast, a time to feast: the crosstalk between metabolism and the circadian clock." *Molecules and Cells* 28:75–80. doi: 10.1007/s10059-009-0113-0.

[7] Brebbia, Robert D., and Kenneth Z. Altshuler. 1965. "Oxygen consumption rate and electroencephalographic stage of sleep." *Science* 1621–3. doi: 10.1126/science.150.3703.1621.

[8] Goldberg, G. R., Prentice, A. M., Davies, H. L., and P. R. Murgatroyd. 1988. "Overnight and basal metabolic rates in men and women." *European Journal of Clinical Nutrition* 42:137–44.

[9] Van Cauter, Eve, Kerkhofs, Myriam, Caufriez, Anne, Van Onderbergen, Anne, Thorner, Michael O., and Georges Copinschi. 1992. "A quantitative estimation of growth hormone secretion in normal man: reproducibility and relation to sleep and time of day." *The Journal of Clinical Endocrinology and Metabolism* 74:1441–50. doi: 10.1210/jcem.74.6.1592892.

[10] Sharma, Sunil, and Mani Kavuru. 2010. "Sleep and metabolism: an overview." *International Journal of Endocrinology* 2010. doi: 10.1155/2010/270832.

[11] Scheen, Andre J., Byrne, Maria M., Plat, Laurence, Leproult, Rachel, and Eve Van Cauter. 1996. "Relationships between sleep quality and glucose regulation in normal humans." *American*

Journal of Physiology 271:E261–70. doi: 10.1152/ajpendo. 1996.271.2.E261.

[12] Morris, Christopher J., Aeschbach, Daniel, and Frank A. J. L. Scheer. 2012. "Circadian system, sleep and endocrinology." *Molecular and Cellular Endocrinology* 349:91–104. doi: 10.1016/j.mce.2011. 09.003.

[13] Peschke, Elmar, and Eckhard Muhlbauer. 2010. "New evidence for a role of melatonin in glucose regulation." *Best practice & research. Clinical endocrinology & metabolism* 24:829–41. doi: 10.1016/j.beem.2010.09.001.

[14] Moller Henry J., and Shirley Lam. 2008. "Quality of life in excessive daytime sleep and hypersomnia." In *Sleep and quality of life in clinical medicine*, edited by Joris Verster, S. R. Pandi-Perumal and David L. Streiner, 107–18.Totowa, NJ: Humana Press.

[15] Heinzer, Raphael, Vat, S., Marques-Vidal P., Marti-Soler, Helena, Andries, D., Tobback, N., Mooser, V., Preisig, M., Malhotra, Atul, Waeber, G., Vollenweider, P., Tafti, Mehdi, and Jose Haba-Rubio. 2015. "Prevalence of sleep-disordered breathing in the general population: the HypnoLaus study." *Lancet Respiratory Medicine* 3:310–8. doi: 10.1016/S2213-2600(15)00043-0.

[16] Raj, Jeffrey P., Hansdak, Samuel G., Naik, Dukhabandhu, Mahendri, Narayani V., and Nihal Thomas. 2019. "SLEep among diabetic patients and their GlycaEmic control (SLEDGE): A pilot observational study." *Journal of Diabetes* 11:122–8. doi: 10.1111/1753-0407.12825.

[17] Lecube, Albert, Sanchez, Enric, Gomez-Peralta, Fernando, Abreu, Cristina, Valls, Joan, Mestre, Olga, Romero, Odile, Martínez, Maria D., Sampol, Gabriel, Ciudin, Andreea, Hernández, Cristina, and Rafael Simó. 2016. "Global Assessment of the Impact of Type 2 Diabetes on Sleep through Specific Questionnaires. A Case-Control Study." *PLoS One* 11:e0157579. doi: 10.1371/journal. pone.0157579.

[18] Raman, Rajiv, Gupta, Aditi, Venkatesh, Kadri, Kulothungan, V aitheeswaran, and Tarun Sharma. 2012. "Abnormal sleep patterns in subjects with type II diabetes mellitus and its effect on diabetic microangiopathies: Sankara Nethralaya Diabetic Retinopathy Epidemiology and Molecular Genetic Study (SN-DREAMS, report 20)." *Acta Diabetologica* 49:255–61. doi: 10.1007/s00592-010-0240-2.

[19] Arosemena Coronel, M., Sanchez Armijos, J., Tettamanti Miranda, D., Vasquez Cedeno, D., Mariani Carrera, R., Navarro Chavez, M., and R. R. Castillo. 2017. "Excessive daytime somnolence is associated with hypoglycemia in adult Latinos with type 2 diabetes mellitus." *Sleep Medicine* 36:6–9. doi: 10.1016/j.sleep.2017.04.012.

[20] Rusu, Adriana, Nita, Cristina, Bala, Cornelia, and Nicolae Hancu. 2011. "Prevalence and predictors of excessive daytime sleepiness in Romanian obese type 2 diabetic patients." *Applied Medical Informatics* 28:41–6.

[21] Obaseki, Daniel O., Kolawole, Babatope A., Gomerep, Simji S., Obaseki, Josephine E., Abidoye, Ibukun A., Ikem, Rosemary T., and Gregory E. Erhabor. 2014. "Prevalence and predictors of obstructive sleep apnea syndrome in a sample of patients with type 2 Diabetes Mellitus in Nigeria." *Nigerian Mededical Journal* 55:24–8. doi: 10.4103/0300-1652.128154.

[22] Johns, Murray W. 1993. "Daytime sleepiness, snoring, and obstructive sleep apnea. The Epworth Sleepiness Scale." *Chest* 103:30–6. doi: 10.1378/chest.103.1.30.

[23] Mitler, Merrill M., Gujavarty, Krishnareddy S., and Carl P. Browman. 1982. "Maintenance of wakefulness test: a polysomnographic technique for evaluation treatment efficacy in patients with excessive somnolence." *Electroencephalography and Clinical Neurophysiology* 53:658–61.

[24] Littner, Michael R., Kushida, Clete, Wise, Merrill, Davila, David G., Morgenthaler, Timothy, Lee-Chiong, Teofilo, Hirshkowitz, Max, Loube, Daniel L., Bailey, Dennis, Berry, Richard B., Kapen, Sheldon, and Milton Kramer; Standards of Practice Committee of

the American Academy of Sleep Medicine. 2005. "Practice parameters for clinical use of the multiple sleep latency test and the maintenance of wakefulness test." *Sleep* 28:113–21. doi: 10.1093/sleep/28.1.113.

[25] Carskadon, Mary A., and William W. Dement. 1982. "The multiple sleep latency test: what does it measure?" *Sleep* 5 Suppl 2:S67–72. doi: 10.1093/sleep/5.s2.s67.

[26] The Report of an American Academy of Sleep Medicine Task Force. 1999. "Sleep-related breathing disorders in adults: recommendations for syndrome definition and measurement techniques in clinical research." *Sleep* 22:667–89. doi: https://doi.org/10.1093/sleep/22.5.667.

[27] Rusu, Adriana, Todea, Doina, Rosca, Loredana, Nita, Cristina, and Cornelia Bala. 2012. "The development of a sleep apnea screening program in Romanian type 2 diabetic patients: a pilot study." *Acta Diabetologica* 49:105–9. doi: 10.1007/s00592-010-0177-5.

[28] Lam, David C., Lui, Macy M., Lam, Jamie C., Ong, Liza H., Lam, Karen S., and Mary S. M. Ip. 2010. "Prevalence and recognition of obstructive sleep apnea in Chinese patients with type 2 diabetes mellitus." *Chest* 138:1101–7. doi: 10.1378/chest.10-0596.

[29] Foster, Gary D., Sanders, Mark H., Millman, Richard, Zammit, Gary, Borradaile, Kelley E., Newman, Anne B., Wadden, Thomas A., Kelley, David, Wing, Rena R., Sunyer, Xavier F., Darcey, Valerie and Samuel T. Kuna; Sleep AHEAD Research Group. 2009. "Obstructive sleep apnea among obese patients with type 2 diabetes." *Diabetes Care* 32:1017–9. doi: 10.2337/dc08-1776.

[30] Laaban, Jean P., Daenen, Simon, Léger, Damien, Pascal, S, Bayon, Virginie, Slama, Gerard, and Fabienne Elgrably. 2009. "Prevalence and predictive factors of sleep apnoea syndrome in type 2 diabetic patients." *Diabetes and Metabolism* 35:372–7. doi: 10.1016/j.diabet.2009.03.007.

[31] Einhorn, Daniel, Stewart, Deirdre A., Erman, Milton K., Gordon, Nancy, Philis-Tsimikas, Athena, and Eileen Casal. 2007.

"Prevalence of sleep apnea in a population of adults with type 2 diabetes mellitus." *Endocrine Practice* 13:355–62. doi: https://doi.org/10.4158/EP.13.4.355.

[32] Rusu, Adriana, Bala, Cornelia G., Craciun, Anca E., and Gabriela Roman. 2017. "HbA1c levels are associated with severity of hypoxemia and not with apnea hypopnea index in patients with type 2 diabetes: Results from a cross-sectional study." *Journal of Diabetes* 9:555–61. doi: 10.1111/1753-0407.12452.

[33] Vgontzas, Alexandros N. 2008. "Excessive daytime sleepiness in sleep apnea: it is not just apnea hypopnea index." *Sleep Medicine* 9:712–4. doi: 10.1016/j.sleep.2008.05.001.

[34] Vgontzas, Alexandros N., Bixler, Edward O., Tan, Tjiauw L., Kantner, Deborah, Martin, Louis F., and Anthony Kales. 1998. "Obesity without sleep apnea is associated with daytime sleepiness." *Archives of Internal Medicine* 158:1333–7. doi:10.1001/archinte.158.
12.1333.

[35] Vgontzas, Alexandros N, Tan, Tjiauw L., Bixler, Edward O., Martin, Louis F., Shubert, Duane, and Anthony Kales.1994. "Sleep apnea and sleep disruption in obese patients." *Archives of Internal Medicine* 154:1705–11. doi:10.1001/archinte.1994.00420150073007.

[36] Roure, Nuria, Gomez, Silvia, Mediano, Olga, Duran, Joaquin, de la Pena, Monica, Capote, Francisco, Teran, Joaquin, Masa, Juan F., Alonso, Maria L., Corral, Jaime, Sánchez-Armengod, Angeles, Martinez, Cristina, Barceló, Antonia, Gozal, David, Marín, Jose M., and Ferran Barbé. 2008. "Daytime sleepiness and polysomnography in obstructive sleep apnea patients." *Sleep Medicine* 9:727–31. doi: 10.1016/j.sleep.2008.02.006.

[37] Romero-Corral, Abel, Caples, Sean M., Lopez-Jimenez, Francisco, and Virend K. Somers. 2010. "Interactions between obesity and obstructive sleep apnea: implications for treatment." *Chest* 137:711–9. doi: 10.1378/chest.09-0360.

[38] Serafini, Francesco M., MacDowell Anderson, W., Rosemurgy, Alexander S., Strait, Tom, and Michel M. Murr. 2001. "Clinical predictors of sleep apnea in patients undergoing bariatric surgery." *Obesity Surgery* 11:28–31. doi: https://doi.org/10.1381/096089201321454079.

[39] Dixon, John B., Schachter, L. M., and P. E. O'Brien. 2005. "Polysomnography before and after weight loss in obese patients with severe sleep apnea." *International Journal of Obesity (Lond).* 29:1048–54. doi: 10.1038/sj.ijo.0802960.

[40] Kingshott, Ruth N., Sime, Patricia J., Engleman, Hather M., and Neil J. Douglas. 1995. "Self assessment of daytime sleepiness: patient versus partner." *Thorax* 50:994–5. doi: 10.1136/thx.50.9.994.

[41] Bixler, Edward O., Vgontzas, Alexandros N., Ten Have, Thomas, Tyson, Kathy, and Anthony Kales. 1998. "Effects of age on sleep apnea in men: I. Prevalence and severity." *American Journal of Respiratory and Critical Care Medicine* 157.144–8. doi: 10.1164/ajrccm.157.1.9706079.

[42] Bixler, Edward O., Vgontzas, Alexandros N., Lin, Hung-Mo, Ten Have, Thomas, Rein, Jennifer, Vela-Bueno, Antonio, and Anthony Kales. 2001. "Prevalence of sleep-disordered breathing in women: effects of gender." *American Journal of Respiratory and Critical Care Medicine* 163:608–13. doi: 10.1164/ajrccm.163.3.9911064.

[43] Young, Terry, Palta, Mari, Dempsey, Jerome, Skatrud, James, Weber, Steven, and Safwan Badr. 1993. "The occurrence of sleep-disordered breathing among middle-aged adults." *The New England Journal of Medicine* 328:1230–5. doi: 10.1056/NEJM199304293281704.

[44] Rusu, Adriana, Nita, Cristina, Todea, Doina, Rosca, Loredana, Bala, Cornelia, and Nicolae Hancu. 2011. "Correlation of the Daytime Sleepiness with Respiratory Sleep Parameters in Patients with Sleep Apnea and Type 2 Diabetes." *Acta Endocrinologica (Bucharest)* 7:163–71. doi: 10.4183/aeb.2011.163.

[45] Pepin, J. L., Viot-Blanc, V., Escourrou, P., Racineux, J. L., Sapene, M., Levy, P., Dervaux, B., Lenne, X., and A. Mallart. 2009.

"Prevalence of residual excessive sleepiness in CPAP-treated sleep apnoea patients: the French multicentre study." *European Respiratory Journal* 33:1062–7. doi: 10.1183/09031936.00016808.

[46] Antic, Nick A., Catcheside, Peter, Buchan, Catherine, Hensley, Michael, Naughton, Matthew T, Rowland, Sharn, Wlliamson, Bernadette, Windler, Samantha, and Doug R. McEvoy. 2011. "The effect of CPAP in normalizing daytime sleepiness, quality of life, and neurocognitive function in patients with moderate to severe OSA." *Sleep* 34:111–9. doi: 10.1093/sleep/34.1.111.

[47] Kara, Belguzar and Ozge Kilic. 2015. "Predictors of poor sleep quality and excessive daytime sleepiness in Turkish adults with type 2 diabetes." *Journal of Clinical Nursing* 24:1436–9. doi: 10.1111/jocn.12710.

[48] Slater, Gemma and Joerg Steier. 2012. "Excessive daytime sleepiness in sleep disorders." *Journal of Thoracic Disease* 4:608–16. doi: 10.3978/j.issn.2072-1439.2012.10.07.

[49] Wang, Fei, Chow, Ines H. I., Li, Lu, Li, Xiao-Hong, Ng, Chee H., Ungvari, Gabor S., Wang, Ai-Hong, Jia, Fu-Jun, Zhang, Ye, and Yu-Tao Xiang. 2019. "Sleep duration and patterns in Chinese patients with diabetes: A meta-analysis of comparative studies and epidemiological surveys." *Perspectives in Psychiatric Care* 55:344–53. doi: 10.1111/ppc.12353.

[50] Mokhlesi, Babak, Temple, Karla A., Tjaden, Ashley H., Edelstein, Sharon L., Utzschneider, Kristina M., Nadeau, Kristen J., Hannon Tamara S., Sam, Susan, Barengolts, Elena, Manchanda, Shalini, Ehrmann, David A., and Eve Van Cauter; RISE Consortium. 2019. "Association of Self-Reported Sleep and Circadian Measures With Glycemia in Adults With Prediabetes or Recently Diagnosed Untreated Type 2 Diabetes." *Diabetes Care* 42:1326–32. doi: 10.2337/dc19-0298.

[51] Tsai, Yi-Wen, Kann, Nai-Hsuan, Tung, Tao-Hsin, Chao, Yi-Jen, Lin, Chin-Jung, Chang, Ko-Chen, Chang, Shy-Shin, and Jau-Yuan Chen. 2012. "Impact of subjective sleep quality on glycemic control

in type 2 diabetes mellitus." *Family Practice* 29:30–5. doi: 10.1093/fampra/cmr041.

[52] Barakat, Safa, Abujbara, Mousa, Banimustafa, Radwan, Batieha, Anwar, and Kamel Ajlouni. 2019. "Sleep Quality in Patients With Type 2 Diabetes Mellitus." *Journal of Clinical Medicine Research* 11:261–6. doi: 10.14740/jocmr2947w.

[53] Cho, Eun-Hee, Lee, HeyJean, Ryu, Ohk H., Choi, Moon G., and Sang-Wood Kim. 2014. "Sleep disturbances and glucoregulation in patients with type 2 diabetes." *Journal of Korean Medical Science* 29:243–7. doi: 10.3346/jkms.2014.29.2.243.

[54] Conway, Silvia G., Roizenblatt, S. S., Palombini, L., Castro, L. S., Bittencourt, L. R., Silva, R. S., and S. Tufik. 2008. "Effect of smoking habits on sleep." *Brazilian Journal of Medical and Biological Research* 41:722–7. doi: 10.1590/s0100-879x2008000800014.

[55] Mooradian, Arshag D. 1988. "Diabetic complications of the central nervous system." *Endocrine Reviews* 9:346–56. doi: 10.1210/edrv-9-3-346.

[56] Khandelwal, Deepak, Dutta, Deep, Chittawar, Sachin, and Sanjay Kalra. 2017. "Sleep Disorders in Type 2 Diabetes." *Indian Journal Endocrinology and Metabolism* 21:758–61. doi: 10.4103/ijem.IJEM_
156_17.

[57] Dixon, John B., Schachter, Linda M., and Paul E. O'Brien. 2001. "Sleep disturbance and obesity: changes following surgically induced weight loss." *Archives of Internal Medicine* 161:102–6. doi:10.1001/archinte.161.1.102.

[58] Mokhber, Somayyeh, Zargham Ravanbakhsh, Paria, Jesmi, Fatemeh, Pishgahroudsari, Mohadeseh, Ghanbari Jolfaei Atefeh, and Abdolreza Pazouki. 2016. "Comparing the Excessive Daytime Sleepiness of Obese and Non-obese Patients." *Iranian Red Crescent Medical Journal* 18:e21964. doi: 10.5812/ircmj.21964.

[59] Fernandez-Mendoza, Julio, Vgontzas, Alexandros N., Kritikou, Ilia, Calhoun, Susan L., Liao, Duanping, and Edward O. Bixler. 2015.

"Natural history of excessive daytime sleepiness: role of obesity, weight loss, depression, and sleep propensity." *Sleep* 38:351–60. doi: 10.5665/sleep.4488.

[60] Theorell-Haglow, Jenny, Akerstedt, Torbjorn, Schwarz, Johanna, and Eva Lindberg. 2015. "Predictors for Development of Excessive Daytime Sleepiness in Women: A Population-Based 10-Year Follow-Up." *Sleep* 38:1995–2003. doi: 10.5665/sleep.5258.

[61] Ng, Winda L., Orellana, Liliana, Shaw, Jonathan E., Wong, Evelyn, and Anna Peeters. 2017. "The relationship between weight change and daytime sleepiness: the Sleep Heart Health Study." *Sleep Medicine* 36:109–18. doi: 10.1016/j.sleep.2017.05.004.

[62] Panossian, Lori A. and Sigrid C. Veasey. 2012. "Daytime sleepiness in obesity: mechanisms beyond obstructive sleep apnea--a review." *Sleep* 35:605–15. doi: 10.5665/sleep.1812.

[63] Varela, Esteban J., Hinojosa, Marcelo W., and Ninh T. Nguyen. 2007. "Resolution of obstructive sleep apnea after laparoscopic gastric bypass." *Obesity Surgery* 17:1279–82. doi: 10.1007/s11695-007-9228-6.

[64] Ng, Winda L., Stevenson, Caroline E., Wong, Evelyn, Tanamas, Stephanie, Boelsen-Robinson, Tara, Shaw, Jonathan E., Naughton, Matthew T., Dixon, John, and Anna Peeters. 2017. "Does intentional weight loss improve daytime sleepiness? A systematic review and meta-analysis." *Obesity Reviews* 18:460–75. doi: 10.1111/obr.12498.

[65] Vgontzas, Alexandros N., Fernandez-Mendoza, Julio, Miksiewicz, Tory, Kritikou, Illia, Shaffer, Michele L., Liao, Duanping, Basta, Maria, and Edward O. Bixler. 2014. "Unveiling the longitudinal association between short sleep duration and the incidence of obesity: the Penn State Cohort." *International Journal of Obesity (Lond)* 38:825–32. doi: 10.1038/ijo.2013.172.

[66] Saper, Clifford B., Fuller, Patrick M., Pedersen, Nigel P., Lu, Jun, and Thomas E. Scammell. 2010. "Sleep state switching." *Neuron* 68:1023–42. doi: 10.1016/j.neuron.2010.11.032.

[67] Sinton, Christopher M., Fitch, Thomas E., and Howard K. Gershenfeld. 1999. "The effects of leptin on REM sleep and slow wave delta in rats are reversed by food deprivation." *Journal of Sleep Research* 8:197–203. doi: https://doi.org/10.1046/j.1365-2869.1999.00158.x|.

[68] Keating, Glenda L., Kuhar, Michael J., Bliwise, Donald L., and David B. Rye. 2010. "Wake promoting effects of cocaine and amphetamine-regulated transcript (CART)." *Neuropeptides* 44:241–6. doi: 10.1016/j.npep.2009.12.013.

[69] Pradhan, Aruna D., Manson, JoAnn, Rifai, Nader, Buring, Julie, and Paul M. Ridker. 2001. "C-reactive protein, interleukin 6, and risk of developing type 2 diabetes mellitus." *JAMA* 286:327–34. doi: 10.1001/jama.286.3.327.

[70] Vgontzas, Alexandros N., Papanicolaou, Dimitris A., Bixler, Edward O., Hopper, Kenneth, Lotsikas, Angela, Lin, Huong-Mo, Kales, Anthony, and George P. Chrousos. 2000. "Sleep apnea and daytime sleepiness and fatigue: relation to visceral obesity, insulin resistance, and hypercytokinemia." *The Journal of Clinical Endocrinology & Metabolism* 85:1151–8. doi: 10.1210/jcem.85.3.6484.

[71] Bauer, Joachim, Hohagen, Fritz, Ebert, T., Timmer, Jens, Ganter, U., Krieger, S., Lis, Stefanie, Postler, E., Voderholzer, Ulrich, and Mathias Berge. 1994. "Interleukin-6 serum levels in healthy persons correspond to the sleep-wake cycle." *The Clinical Investigator* 72:315. doi: https://doi.org/10.1007/BF00180048.

[72] Sothern, Robert B., Roitman-Johnson, B., Kanabrocki, E. L., Yager, J. G., Fuerstenberg, Richard K., Weatherbee, J. A., Young, M. R., Nemchausky, B. M., and L. E. Scheving. 1995. "Circadian characteristics of interleukin-6 in blood and urine of clinically healthy men." *In Vivo* 9:331–9.

[73] Gudewill, Susanne, Pollmacher, Thomas, Vedder, Helmut, Schreiber, Wolfgang, Fassbender, Klaus, and Florian Holsboer. 1992. "Nocturnal plasma levels of cytokines in healthy men."

European Archives of Psychiatry and Clinical Neuroscience 242:53–6. doi: https://doi.org/10.1007/BF02190343.

[74] Vgontzas, Alexandros N., Papanicolaou, Dimitris A., Bixler, Edward O., Kales, Anthony, Tyson, Kathy, and George P. Chrousos. 1997. "Elevation of plasma cytokines in disorders of excessive daytime sleepiness: role of sleep disturbance and obesity." *Journal of Clinical Endocrinology & Metabolism* 82:1313–6. doi: 10.1210/jcem.82.5.
3950.

[75] Vgontzas, Alexandros N., Zoumakis, Emmanouil, Lin, Hung-Mo, Bixler, Edward O., Trakada, Georgia, and George P. Chrousos. 2004. "Marked decrease in sleepiness in patients with sleep apnea by etanercept, a tumor necrosis factor-alpha antagonist." *Journal of Clinical Endocrinology & Metabolism* 89:4409–13. doi: 10.1210/jc.2003-031929.

[76] Opp, Mark R., Kapas, Levente, and Linda A. Toth. 1992. "Cytokine involvement in the regulation of sleep." *Proceedings of the Society for Experimental Biology and Medicine* 201:16–27. doi: 10.3181/00379727-201-43474.

[77] Moldofsky, Harvey, Lue, Franklin A., Eisen, J., Keystone, Edward, and Reginald M. Gorczynski. 1986. "The relationship of interleukin-1 and immune functions to sleep in humans." *Psychosomatic Medicine* 48:309–18.

[78] Kapas, Levente, Hong, Lielie, Cady, Alan B., Opp, Mark R., Postlethwaite, Arnold E., Seyer, Jerome M., and James M. Krueger. 1992. "Somnogenic, pyrogenic, and anorectic activities of tumor necrosis factor-alpha and TNF-alpha fragments." *American Journal of Physiology* 263:R708–15. doi: 10.1152/ajpregu.1992.263.3.R708.

[79] Stephens, Jacqueline M., Lee, Jongsoon, and Paul F. Pilch. 1997 "Tumor necrosis factor-alpha-induced insulin resistance in 3T3-L1 adipocytes is accompanied by a loss of insulin receptor substrate-1 and GLUT4 expression without a loss of insulin receptor-mediated signal transduction." *Journal of Biological Chemistry* 272:971–6. doi: 10.1074/jbc.272.2.971.

[80] Wellen, Kathryn E., and Gokhan S. Hotamisligil. 2005 "Inflammation, stress, and diabetes." *The Journal of Clinical Investigation* 115:1111–9. doi: 10.1172/JCI25102.

[81] Fasshauer, Mathias, and Ralf Paschke. 2003. "Regulation of adipocytokines and insulin resistance." *Diabetologia* 46:1594–603. doi: 10.1007/s00125-003-1228-z.

[82] Hotamisligil, Gokhan S. 2008. "Inflammation and endoplasmic reticulum stress in obesity and diabetes." *Internationa Journal of Obesity (Lond)* 32 Suppl 7:S52–4. doi: 10.1038/ijo.2008.238.

[83] Calle, Mariana C., and Maria-Luz Fernandez. 2012. "Inflammation and type 2 diabetes." *Diabetes & Metabolism* 38:183–91. doi: 10.1016/j.diabet.2011.11.006.

[84] Alvarez, Carlos E., and Gregor J. Sutcliffe. 2002. "Hypocretin is an early member of the incretin gene family." *Neuroscience Letters* 324:169–72. doi: 10.1016/s0304-3940(02)00195-7.

[85] Tsujino, Natsuko, and Takeshi Sakurai. 2009. "Orexin/hypocretin: a neuropeptide at the interface of sleep, energy homeostasis, and reward system." *Pharmacological Reviews* 61:162–76. doi: 10.1124/pr.109.001321.

[86] Cai, Xue J., Widdowson, Peter S., Harrold, Joanne, Wilson, Shelag, Buckingham, Robin E., Arch, Jonathan R. S., Tadayyon, Mohammad, Clapham, John C., Wilding, John, and Gareth Williams. 1999. "Hypothalamic orexin expression: modulation by blood glucose and feeding." *Diabetes* 48:2132–7. doi: 10.2337/diabetes.48.11.2132.

[87] Sakurai, Takeshi, Amemiya, Akira, Ishii, Makoto, Matsuzaki, Ichiyo, Chemelli, Richard M., Tanaka, Hirokazu, Williams, Clay S., Richardson, James A., Kozlowski, Gerald P., Wilson, Shelagh, Arch, Jonathan R. S., Buckingham, Robin E., Haynes, Andrea C., Carr, Steven A., Annan, Roland S., McNulty, Dean E., Liu, Wu-Schyong, Terrett, Jonathan A., Elshourbagy, Nabil A., Bergsma, Derk J., and Masashi Yanagisawa. 1998. "Orexins and orexin receptors: a family of hypothalamic neuropeptides and G protein-

coupled receptors that regulate feeding behavior." *Cell* 92:573–85. doi: 10.1016/s0092-8674(02)09256-5.

[88] Pedrazzoli, Mario, D'Almeida, Vania, Martins, Paulo J. F., Machado, Ricardo B., Ling, Lin, Nishino, Seiji, Tufik, Sergio, and Emmanuel Mignot. 2004. Increased hypocretin-1 levels in cerebrospinal fluid after REM sleep deprivation. *Brain Research* 995:1–6. doi: 10.1016/j.brainres.2003.09.032.

[89] Castillo, Pablo R., Mignot, Emmanuel, Woodruff, Bryan K., and Bradley F. Boeve. 2004. "Undetectable CSF hypocretin-1 in "Hashimoto's encephalopathy" associated with coma." *Neurology* 62:1909. doi: 10.1212/01.wnl.0000125284.19326.80.

[90] Burdakov, Denis, and Haris Alexopoulos. 2005. "Metabolic state signalling through central hypocretin/orexin neurons." *Journal of Cellular and Molecular Medicine* 9:795–803. doi: 10.1111/j.1582-4934.2005.tb00380.x.

[91] Burdakov, Denis, Gerasimenko, Oleg, and Alexei Verkhratsky. 2005. "Physiological changes in glucose differentially modulate the excitability of hypothalamic melanin-concentrating hormone and orexin neurons in situ." *The Journal of Neuroscience* 25:2429–33. doi: 10.1523/JNEUROSCI.4925-04.2005.

[92] Williams, Rhiannan H., Alexopoulos, Haris, Jensen, Lise T., Fugger, Lars, and Denis Burdakov. 2008. "Adaptive sugar sensors in hypothalamic feeding circuits." *Proceedings of the National Academy of Sciences of the United States of America* 105:11975–80. doi: 10.1073/pnas.0802687105.

[93] Idris, Iskandar, Abdulla, Haitham, Tilbrook, Sean, Dean, Roy, and Nabeel Ali. 2013. "Exenatide improves excessive daytime sleepiness and wakefulness in obese patients with type 2 diabetes without obstructive sleep apnoea." *Journal of Sleep Research* 22:70–5. doi: 10.1111/j.1365-2869.2012.01030.x.

[94] Acuna-Goycolea, Claudio, and Anthony van den Pol. 2004. "Glucagon-like peptide 1 excites hypocretin/orexin neurons by direct and indirect mechanisms: implications for viscera-mediated

arousal." *The Journal of Neuroscience* 24:8141–52. doi: 10.1523/JNEUROSCI.1607-04.2004.

[95] Roy, Tapash, and Cathy E. Lloyd. 2012. "Epidemiology of depression and diabetes: a systematic review." *Journal of Affective Disorders* 142 Suppl:S8–21. doi: 10.1016/S0165-0327(12)70004-6.

[96] Baumeister, Harald, Hutter, Nico, Bengel, Jurgen, and Martin Harter. 2011. "Quality of life in medically ill persons with comorbid mental disorders: a systematic review and meta-analysis." *Psychotherapy and Psychosomatics* 80:275–86. doi: 10.1159/000323404.

[97] Gonzalez, Jeffrey S., Peyrot, Mark, McCarl, Lauren A., Collins, Erin M., Serpa, Luis, Mimiaga, Matthew J., and Steven A. Safren. 2008. "Depression and diabetes treatment nonadherence: a meta-analysis." *Diabetes Care* 31:2398–403. doi: 10.2337/dc08-1341.

[98] Egede, Leonard E., Nietert, Paul J., and Deyi Zheng. 2005. "Depression and all-cause and coronary heart disease mortality among adults with and without diabetes." *Diabetes Care* 28:1339–45. doi: 10.2337/diacare.28.6.1339.

[99] American Psychiatric Association. 2013. *Diagnostic and statistical manual of mental disorders DSM-5. Fifth edition.* Arlington: American Psychiatric Association Publishing.

[100] Bixler, Edward O., Vgontzas, Alexandros N., Lin, Hung-Mo, Calhoun, Susan L., Vela-Bueno, Antonio, and Anthony Kales. 2005. "Excessive daytime sleepiness in a general population sample: the role of sleep apnea, age, obesity, diabetes, and depression." *The Journal of Clinical Endocrinology & Metabolism* 90:4510–5. doi: 10.1210/jc.2005-0035.

[101] Koutsourelakis, Ioannis, Perraki, Eleni, Bonakis, Anastasios, Vagiakis, Emmanouil, Roussos, Charis, and Spyros Zakynthinos. 2008. "Determinants of subjective sleepiness in suspected obstructive sleep apnoea." *Journal of Sleep Research* 17:437–43. doi: 10.1111/j.1365-2869.2008.00663.x.

[102] Dixon, John B., Dixon, Maureen E., Anderson, Margaret L., Schachter, Linda, and Paul E. O'Brien. 2007. "Daytime sleepiness in

the obese: not as simple as obstructive sleep apnea." *Obesity (Silver Spring)* 15:2504–11. doi: 10.1038/oby.2007.297.

[103] Medeiros, Camila, Bruin, Veralice, Ferrer, Debora, Paiva, Ticiana, Montenegro Junior, Renan, Forti, Adriana, and Pedro Bruin. 2013. "Excessive daytime sleepiness in type 2 diabetes." *Arquivos Brasileiros de Endocrinologia & Metabologia* 57:425–30. doi: http://dx.doi.org/10.1590/S0004-27302013000600003

[104] Jacobs, Barry L., and Dennis J. McGinty. 1971. "Effects of food deprivation on sleep and wakefulness in the rat." *Experimental Neurolurology* 30:212–22. doi: https://doi.org/10.1016/S0014-4886(71)80002-X.

[105] Danguir, Jaber, and Stylianos Nicolaidis. 1979. "Dependence of sleep on nutrients' availability." *Physiology & Behavior* 22:735–40. doi: https://doi.org/10.1016/0031-9384(79)90240-3.

[106] Gais, Steffen, Born, Jan, Peters, Achim, Schultes, Bernd, Heindl, Britta, Fehm, Horst L., and Kern Werner. 2003. "Hypoglycemia counterregulation during sleep." *Sleep* 26:55–9. doi: 10.1093/sleep/26.1.55.

[107] Danguir, Jaber. 1987. "Cafeteria diet promotes sleep in rats." *Appetite* 8:49–53. doi: https://doi.org/10.1016/S0195-6663(87) 80026-0.

[108] Harnish, Michael J., Greenleaf, Shelley R., and William C. Orr. 1998. "A comparison of feeding to cephalic stimulation on postprandial sleepiness." *Physiology & Behavior* 64:93–6. doi: 10.1016/s0031-9384(98)00025-0.

[109] Craig, Angus, and Eileen Richardson. 1989. "Effects of experimental and habitual lunch-size on performance, arousal, hunger and mood." *International Archives of Occupational and Environmental Health* 61:313–9.

[110] Wells, Anita S., Read, Nicholas W., and Angus Craig. 1995. "Influences of dietary and intraduodenal lipid on alertness, mood, and sustained concentration." *British Journal of Nutrition* 74:115–23. doi: https://doi.org/10.1079/BJN19950111.

[111] Wells, Anita S., Read, Nicholas W., Idzikowski, Chris, and Jane Jones. 1998. "Effects of meals on objective and subjective measures of daytime sleepiness." *Journal of Applied Physiology* 84:507–15. doi: 10.1152/jappl.1998.84.2.507.

[112] Orr, William C., Shadid, Gregory, Harnish, Michael J., and Sigrid Elsenbruch. 1997. "Meal composition and its effect on postprandial sleepiness." *Physiology & Behavior* 62:709–12. doi: 10.1016/s0031-9384(97)00012-7.

[113] Wells, Anita S., Read, Nicholas W., Uvnas-Moberg, Kerstin, and Pawel Alster. 1997. "Influences of fat and carbohydrate on postprandial sleepiness, mood, and hormones." *Physiology & Behavior* 61:679-86. doi: 10.1016/s0031-9384(96)00519-7.

[114] Hansen, Michael K., Taishi, Ping, Chen, Zutang, and James M. Krueger. 1998. "Cafeteria feeding induces interleukin-1beta mRNA expression in rat liver and brain." *American Journal of Physiology* 274:R1734–9. doi: 10.1152/ajpregu.1998.274.6.R1734.

[115] Hansen, Michael K., Kapas, Levente, Fang, Jidong, and James M. Krueger. 1998. "Cafeteria diet-induced sleep is blocked by subdiaphragmatic vagotomy in rats." *American Journal of Physiology* 274:R168–74. doi: 10.1152/ajpregu.1998.274.1.R168.

[116] Lopes, Tassia V. C., Borba, Matheus E. S., Lopes, Raissa V. C., Fisberg, Regina M., Paim, Samantha L., Teodoro, Vinicius V., Zimberg, Ioan Z., Araújo, Lucio B., Shivappa, Nitin, Hébert, James R., and Cibele A. Crispim. 2019. "Association between the inflammatory potential of the diet and sleep parameters in sleep apnea patients." *Nutrition* 66:5–10. doi: 10.1016/j.nut.2019.04.003.

[117] Lehrskov, Louise L., Dorph, Emma, Widmer, Andrea M., Hepprich, Matthias, Siegenthaler, Judith, Timper, Katharina, and Marc Y. Donath. 2018. "The role of IL-1 in postprandial fatigue." *Molecular Metabolism* 12:107–12. doi: 10.1016/j.molmet.2018.04.001.

[118] Vasconcelos, Joao P., Medeiros da Costa Daniele, Thiago, Carvalhedo de Bruin, Pedro F., Costa e Forti, Adriana, and Veralice Meireles Sales de bruin V. 2016. "Daytime sleepiness in patients with type 2 Diabetes Mellitus – a prospective cohort study."

International Archives of Medicine 9: Accessed July, 12, 2019. http://imed.pub/ojs/index.php/iam/article/view/1827. doi: 10.3823/2099.

[119] Iftikhar, Imran H., Kline, Christopher E., and Shawn D. Youngstedt. 2014. "Effects of exercise training on sleep apnea: a meta-analysis." *Lung* 192:175–84. doi: 10.1007/s00408-013-9511-3.

[120] Chasens, Eileen R., Umlauf, Mary G., and Terri E. Weaver. 2009. "Sleepiness, physical activity, and functional outcomes in veterans with type 2 diabetes." *Applied Nursing Research* 22:176–82. doi: 10.1016/j.apnr.2007.12.001.

[121] Thomas, Naveena, Alder, Elizabeth, and Graham P. Leese. 2004. "Barriers to physical activity in patients with diabetes." *Postgraduate Medical Journal* 80:287–91. doi: 10.1136/pgmj.2003.010553.

[122] Duclos, Martine, Dejager, Sylvie, Postel-Vinay, Nicolas, di Nicola, Sylvie, Quere, Stephane, and Beatrice Fiquet. 2015. "Physical activity in patients with type 2 diabetes and hypertension--insights into motivations and barriers from the MOBILE study." *Vascular Health and Risk Management* 11:361–71. doi: 10.2147/VHRM.S84832.

[123] Maluf, Katrina S., and Michael J. Mueller. 2003. "Novel Award 2002. Comparison of physical activity and cumulative plantar tissue stress among subjects with and without diabetes mellitus and a history of recurrent plantar ulcers." *Clinical Biomechanics* 18:567–75. doi: https://doi.org/10.1016/S0268-0033(03)00118-9.

[124] Inkster, Berit, Riha, Renata L., Van Look, Liesbeth, Williamson, Rachel, McLachlan, Stela, Frier, Brian M., Strachan, Mark W. J., Price, Jackie F., and Rebecca M. Reynolds. 2013. "Association between excessive daytime sleepiness and severe hypoglycemia in people with type 2 diabetes: the Edinburgh Type 2 Diabetes Study." *Diabetes Care* 36:4157–9. doi: 10.2337/dc13-0863.

[125] Bloomfield, Hanna E., Greer, Nancy, Newman, David, MacDonald, Roderick, Carlyle, Maureen, Fitzgerald, Patrick, Rutks, Indulis, and Timothy J. Wilt. 2012. *Predictors and Consequences of Severe*

Hypoglycemia in Adults with Diabetes – A Systematic Review of the Evidence. VA-ESP Project #09-009. Accessed July, 14 2019. https://www.ncbi.nlm.nih.gov/books/NBK114893/pdf/Bookshelf_NBK114893.pdf.

[126] Aung, Phyu P., Strachan, Mark W., Frier, Brian M., Butcher, Isabella, Deary, Ian J., and Jackie F. Price; Edinburgh Type 2 Diabetes Study Investigators. 2012. "Severe hypoglycaemia and late-life cognitive ability in older people with Type 2 diabetes: the Edinburgh Type 2 Diabetes Study." *Diabetic Medicine* 29:328–36. doi: 10.1111/j.1464-5491.2011.03505.x.

[127] Johnston, Stephen S., Conner, Christopher, Aagren, Mark, Smith, David M., Bouchard, Jonathan, and Jason Brett. 2011. "Evidence linking hypoglycemic events to an increased risk of acute cardiovascular events in patients with type 2 diabetes." *Diabetes Care* 34:1164–70. doi: 10.2337/dc10-1915.

[128] Lo, Shih-Chang, Yang, Yi-Sun, Kornelius, Edy, Huang, Jing-Yang, Lai, Yung-Rung, Huang, Chien-Ning, and Jen-Yuan Chiou. 2019. "Early cardiovascular risk and all-cause mortality following an incident of severe hypoglycaemia: *A population-based cohort study." Diabetes Obesity and Metabolism* 21:1878–1885. doi: 10.1111/dom.13746.

[129] Keskin, Ahmet, Unalacak, Murat, Bilge, Ugur, Yildiz, Pinar, Guler, Seda, Selcuk, Engin B., and Muzaffer Bilgin. 2015. "Effects of Sleep Disorders on Hemoglobin A1c Levels in Type 2 Diabetic Patients." *Chinese Medical Journal (Engl)* 128:3292–7. doi: 10.4103/0366-6999.171415.

[130] Czeisler, Charles A. 2011. "Impact of sleepiness and sleep deficiency on public health--utility of biomarkers." *Journal of Clinical Sleep Medicine* 7(5 Suppl):S6–8. doi: 10.5664/JCSM.1340.

[131] Chasens, Eileen R., Korytkowski, Mary, Sereika, Susan M., and Lora E. Burke. 2013. "Effect of poor sleep quality and excessive daytime sleepiness on factors associated with diabetes self-management." *The Diabetes Educator* 39:74–82. doi: 10.1177/0145721712467683.

In: New Research on Sleep …
Editor: Olivier Ratté
ISBN: 978-1-53616-882-2

Chapter 2

Sleep Dysfunction in the Critically Ill

***Joey Carlin*[1]*, Carl Boethel*[1]*, Shekhar Ghamande*[1] *and Salim Surani*[1,2]**
[1]Division of Pulmonary, Critical Care and Sleep Medicine,
Baylor Scott and White Health, Temple, TX, US
[2]Division of Pulmonary and Critical Care,
Corpus Christi Medical Center, Corpus Christi, TX, US

Abstract

Disruption of sleep in critically ill patients occurs through four mechanisms; decreased total sleep time, alteration of sleep architecture, disturbance of circadian rhythm and fragmentation of sleep. Sleep dysfunction has multiple causes in critically ill patients, some of which are extrinsic to the patient (e.g., a bright and noisy ICU environment), and some which are intrinsic to the patient (e.g., the patient's own underlying illness). Common therapeutic interventions utilized in many critically ill patients, such as common ICU medications and mechanical ventilation, can exacerbate sleep disruption. Disruption of sleep can further destabilize a patient or complicate their ICU course. Simple interventions are important to implement to halt this feedback loop and improve a patient's sleep. Even after recovery, patients are at risk for long-term disruption of healthy sleep due to their prior critical illness.

Keywords: sleep, dysfunction, sleep time, sleep architecture, circadian rhythm, fragmentation of sleep, critical care, ICU, environment, polysomnography

INTRODUCTION

"To die, to sleep – to sleep, perchance to dream – ay, there's the rub, for in this sleep of death what dreams may come…"
– William Shakespeare, Hamlet.

Poor sleep quality is one of the leading sources of anxiety and stress in intensive care unit patients; it is a possible cause of delirium, reduced immune and metabolic function and respiratory dysfunction [1, 2]. Critically ill patients suffer from fragmented sleep, disrupted circadian rhythms and abnormal sleep architecture.

The therapeutic milieu of the ICU is a bright, noisy environment with frequent patient-care interactions throughout each night. The ICU environment contributes significantly to sleep disturbance, but is not the sole culprit. Critical illness causes physiologic changes that disrupt the sleep-promoting neural pathways, and many common ICU medications cause changes in sleep architecture in addition to insomnia.

Patients who have higher acuity illnesses have more pronounced disruption of their sleep, [3] especially if they require vasopressor support or mechanical ventilation [4]. Patients on mechanical ventilation have a unique, constant, unnatural stimulus that can lead to frequent arousals. These extremes are more obvious in their detriment to natural sleep, but lab draws and simple interventions like adjusting IV drips and administering medications contribute to frequent arousals in this setting [5].

Increasingly providers are becoming aware of how dissimilar this setting is to an ideal home sleep environment and the negative effect this has on circadian rhythms and sleep architecture and by extension, how that negatively impacts the recovery of the critically ill. A growing area of research focuses on improving sleep quality in this vulnerable population without sacrificing the safety and quality of care provided at night in an intensive care unit.

Sleep Architecture and Circadian Rhythm

Disruption of sleep in critically ill patients occurs through four mechanisms; decreased total sleep time, alteration of sleep architecture, disturbance of circadian rhythm, and fragmentation of sleep [1]. Each of these individually can lead to somnolence and development of complications of sleep deprivation, but in concert their impact can be profound. These effects are seen both in medical and surgical critically ill populations [6, 7] and become more pronounced as acuity of illness worsens [3].

Sleep duration is markedly decreased in the ICU population compared to the needs of a healthy person. This is in contrast to what we would expect for their natural needs during this time; when people become ill their bodies trigger signals through cytokines which can stimulate increased somnolence [8]. One study of nine surgical intensive care unit patients found that the mean total sleep time for the first 48 hours after admission was less than two hours per day [6]. This same group of patients also demonstrated concomitant alterations in their sleep architecture. They had reduced REM sleep (9.3% of time compared to healthy controls) and markedly reduced levels of stage 3 sleep (5.9% of time compared to healthy controls). Several patients in the cohort did not achieve any REM sleep during their first 48 hours in the ICU. In contrast, a study of 20 mechanically ventilated adults with ARDS in the medical ICU who underwent 24-hour PSG found three distinct patterns, all of which were abnormal [4]. The first group (8/20 patients) had the lightest sedation; they had highly fragmented sleep with an average 4.0 hours spent sleeping during the day and 3.0 hours spent sleeping at night. In this group patients spent roughly an equal time in non-REM and REM sleep. The second two groups had deeper sedation and more total sleep time. The second group (5/20 patients) had atypical sleep which alternated between stage 1 and stage 3 sleep, with no stage 2 and markedly reduced REM sleep. The third group (7/20 patients) were termed to be the "coma" group; their sleep had more than 50% of delta or theta activity on EEG and the majority of these patients did not show any EEG activity in response to deep painful stimuli.

Loss of normal sleep architecture may have profound consequences.

Stage 3 sleep is the most restorative stage of sleep; NREM sleep is thought to be when the body coordinates repairing tissues and boosting the immune system. This is thought to be part of the reason illness triggers cytokines that increase sleep time and slow wave sleep. The other phase that is decreased in critically ill patients is REM sleep; this phase of sleep is important for consolidation of memory. Gaps in memory from ICU stay are thought to contribute to delirium and long-term PTSD secondary to a patient's critical illness.

Circadian rhythm disruption and fragmentation of sleep both appear to be nearly universal in the ICU. One study of MICU patients found that of 22 patients (of which 20 were mechanically ventilated), all studied patients had circadian abnormalities and fragmented sleep [7]. While the mean total sleep time was 8.8 hours for their cohort, patients had a mean number of 41 sleep periods per day with a mean sleep length of 15 minutes per sleep period. In their cohort 57% of patient's total sleep time occurred during the day and 43% at night. Sedation level with intermittent lorazepam or intermittent fentanyl did not appear to prevent fragmentation of sleep in this study.

Critically ill patients appear to have decreased total sleep time, alteration of sleep architecture, disturbance of circadian rhythm, and fragmentation of sleep occurring together in the majority of patients over a 24-hour period. This observation supports the theory that sleep deprivation in the ICU is multifactorial, and its improvement will most likely require a multisystem approach.

FACTORS IMPACTING SLEEP IN CRITICAL CARE

Intrinsic Factors: Critical Illness, Pain, Stress, and History

In addition to factors that are extrinsic to the patient (such as the noise and brightness of an ICU room), several important intrinsic factors impact the quality of sleep of critically ill patients. In a comparison study in which healthy volunteers served as controls, the critically ill patients had less total sleep time and less slow wave sleep [5].

Critical illness encephalopathy can independently disrupt a patient's normal sleep-wake cycle through inflammation. The cytokines interleukin-1 beta and tumor necrosis factor alpha both promote somnolence and increase REM sleep under normal physiologic conditions [9]. Under physiologic stress, these same cytokines play a critical role in host protection, with both IL-1 and TNF-alpha levels rising and then promoting rest in the host patient.

Metabolic derangement from sepsis, hypotension and a number of other factors can directly alter the sleep wake balance. Improvement in mental status can lag behind resolution of the inciting factor. Critical illness itself is a risk factor for sleep disturbance that can only be modified by appropriately treating the underlying cause.

Both pain and anxiety can cause insomnia and contribute to sleep fragmentation [10]. It is important to address these factors and understand the effects that many of the common medications used to address these symptoms have on a patient's sleep.

Patients with a prior history of insomnia and patients who use sleep aids regularly at home prior to admission to the hospital are at higher risk for development of sleep disturbances in the ICU [10]. While this can help identify critically ill patients at higher risk for developing sleep related complications there are not currently any recommendations specific to these patients to reduce dysfunctional sleep.

The Impact of the ICU Environment on Sleep

Noise

Minimizing noise has a historic role in establishing a therapeutic milieu; Florence Nightingale, an early nursing pioneer of quality improvement who came to fame during the Crimean war once wrote, "Unnecessary noise is the most cruel abuse of care which can be inflicted on either the sick or the well." Despite the common knowledge of the potential harm nocturnal noise can have, the ICU is not a quiet place at night. One study of 22 patients in the medical ICU (20 on mechanical ventilation) over 24-48 hours with multiple environmental monitors and polysomnography attributed 17% of arousals to elevated sound levels [7].

The World Health Organization (WHO) released guidelines on noise pollution in a document titled *Guidelines for Community Noise*; this included recommendations for noise levels in hospitals. The recommendation was that average noise levels should not exceed 35 decibels, and that maximum levels should not exceed 40 decibels [11]. The United States Environmental Protection agency has echoed these guidelines, recommending that sound levels should not exceed 45 decibels during the day or 35 decibels at night [12]. Sound levels of 40 decibels correspond to level of sound of the hum of a refrigerator [13].

One study of overnight noise in the ICU found peaks of 85 decibels or higher occurred 12 times an hour on average between 9 PM and 6AM [14]. For comparison, a washing machine emits sound around 70 decibels and urban road traffic has sound levels of 80-85 decibels [13]. Polysomnography performed on patients in the ICU has shown that noises above 80 decibels are associated with arousals from sleep [15]. One study of healthy volunteers exposed to simulated ICU sounds while sleeping overnight in a sleep lab found volunteers had increased sleep latency, frequent arousals, and decreased total REM sleep [16]. Efforts to decrease peak noise levels in the ICU have had limited success; one trial that instituted a multipronged intervention was able to reduce events where noise levels were above 60 decibels from an average of 1735 events down to 1289 in a 24 hour period, however this had little effect on the average noise level (53.8 decibels compared to 54.2 decibels, $p = 0.96$) and no significant clinical effect [17].

Patient Care Activities

Critically ill patients require frequent interventions during the stabilization phase that unfortunately can contribute to recurrent nightly arousals. Lab draws, neurologic checks, finger stick glucose monitoring, and routine daily baths are often scheduled throughout the night. Procedures and imaging frequently cannot be delayed until morning and have to be performed at the expense of patients' rest. In one study, patients had an average of 42.6 interactions with ICU staff over the course of a night, with higher acuity correlating with more interventions during normal sleep hours [18]. Patients in this study only had a 6% chance of having 2 or more continuous hours of sleep without interruption.

In contrast to the perception that noise and caregiver interaction were at fault for the constant sleep disruption, another study utilizing 24-hour polysomnography with time-synchronized environment monitoring found that patients had an average of 7.8 patient care activities per hour of sleep, but that these events only caused 7.1% of the total arousals from sleep [4]. Both noise and patient care activities together were associated with less than 30% of total arousals, suggesting that these two factors that historically have received the most blame for sleep disturbance were only part of a larger complex puzzle.

Nocturnal Light Levels

Overnight light in the ICU contributes to sleep disturbance. Light levels as low as 100 lux stimulate melatonin, and levels as low as 300 lux disrupt the circadian pacemaker [19]. The rooms of patients in the ICU have levels up to 1000 lux [20].

The difficulty here lies in balancing the need for staff being able to safely perform patient evaluations and patient care interactions with minimizing abnormal light exposure. Much of the light exposure is directly tied to points when staff are directly interacting with patients, which was reflected by reports of ICU survivors that light did not disturb them as much as patient care interventions and noise [21].

Mechanical Ventilation

Patients on mechanical ventilation experience continuous unnatural stimuli which is reflected by severe abnormalities in sleep. Ventilator dysynchrony increased during NREM sleep leading to marked sleep fragmentation with over 20 arousals per hour on average [4, 22].

Mechanical ventilation can also increase a patient's risk for apneas. Patients who are maintained on pressure support ventilation have increased rates of central apneas. [1] Pressure support ventilation is also associated with a higher number of arousals compared to assist control ventilation [23]. This is thought to be due to higher minute ventilation with decreased CO_2 levels that can potentiate central apneas and lead to arousals from sleep. This is one hypothetical reason why it may be safer to maintain patients on volume or pressure control overnight even if patients have tolerated pressure support during the daytime.

Sleep Disruption by Common Medications Used in the Critically Ill

Many of the medications that are commonly required to stabilize patients affect sleep. Some of these medications cause insomnia, others affect the architecture of sleep. In many cases, despite these known side effects, there simply are not better alternatives at this time and clinicians have to prioritize stabilizing patients over downstream consequences.

Sedatives

While sedatives can improve sleep efficiency and increase total sleep time, this is at the cost of stage 3 and REM sleep [24]. Propofol, an agent commonly used in the ICU for deep continuous sedation for ventilated patients, has been implicated as a REM suppressant that causes poor reported sleep quality and delirium [25]. Benzodiazepines, commonly used for deep continuous sedation or intermittent sedation, are implicated in REM sleep suppression. Their discontinuation has been found to cause rebound insomnia, which most likely occurs due to use-dependent downregulation of GABA receptors [26] The alpha-2 agonist dexmedetomidine, which has sedative and anxiolytic effects, causes less alteration on natural sleep architecture compared to other sedative agents [25]. However, the clinical implications of this finding need to be further studied. Unfortunately, despite increasing sleep time and reducing sleep fragmentation, excessive sedation increases ICU delirium and increases the risk of developing post-ICU syndrome (a condition seen in many survivors of critical illness where patients can have a combination of physical, psychiatric or cognitive impairment). Regardless of a potential benefit to sleep sedatives should be minimized whenever clinically appropriate.

Analgesics

The effect of treating pain in critically ill patients requires finding a delicate balance. Undertreated pain will lead to sleep fragmentation and worsening delirium, but both opiate and non-opiate pain medications can disturb sleep. Opiates reduce stage 3 and REM sleep and induce central sleep apnea [27]. NSAID medications are noted to increase sleep fragmentation and delay onset of deep sleep stages [28]. The effect of NSAIDS on sleep has been attributed to inhibition of prostaglandin synthesis along with suppression of melatonin secretion and effects on body temperature. Acetaminophen, an analgesic which is rarely sufficient to fully control pain in critically ill patients when used alone, but it is often used in combination with other analgesics. The effects on sleep architecture show disruption of sleep stages on overnight polysomnogram and implication of worsening subjective sleep [28]. Despite all of this, leaving a patient in uncontrolled pain will also lead to sleep fragmentation, loss of deep sleep, worsened subjective measures of rest and delirium. The onus is on the clinician to find the appropriate balance when treating a patient's pain.

Antipsychotics

Antipsychotic medications are used extensively in the ICU to treat delirium. While a recent study has called into question the efficacy of these medications, [29] they remain a highly utilized class of medications. Both typical and atypical antipsychotic medications improve sleep efficiency and increase slow wave sleep through antagonism of histamine H1 receptors [30]. While both types of antipsychotics are sedating, atypical antipsychotics (e.g., quetiapine and olanzapine) are more so than typical antipsychotics (e.g haloperidol) [31].

There are no studies that examine the effects of these drugs in critically ill patients, but there is one trial where healthy subjects were given olanzapine, risperidone or haloperidol [32]. Patients who received olanzapine or risperidone had increased stage 3 and REM sleep with improved sleep efficiency. Patients who received haloperidol had increased N2 sleep without loss of stage 3 or REM sleep.

Corticosteroids

Corticosteroids are known to cause insomnia. Steroid use reduces REM sleep and causes increased sleep fragmentation in non-critically ill patients [33]. The benefits seen with the use of the APROCCHUS and ADRENAL studies have shown that steroids can have a positive effect on septic shock patients. Though the amount of increase in steroid use in this setting is unknown, the must assume that usage has increased. While the effect of corticosteroids on sleep has not been studied in this population, the presumption is that they lead to worsened insomnia, sleep fragmentation and thus delirium, however this link is not proven.

Respiratory Medication

While agitation and insomnia can be caused by beta-agonists, [26] agitation and insomnia also can be caused by respiratory distress. Overall this is a class of medications whose benefits to sleep likely outweigh the potential harm.

Cardiovascular Medications

Vasopressors and Inotropes are vital in the treatment of patients in shock. Both of these classes of medications have been implicated in development of insomnia through stimulation of adrenergic receptors [1]. One study evaluated surgical ICU patients after esophagectomy and analyzed risk for post-operative insomnia; sleep disturbance was independently predicted by duration of dopamine infusions in their cohort [34]. These medications also have been shown to reduce stage 3 and REM sleep [26].

Atrial fibrillation is the most common arrhythmia in critically ill patients [35]. Critical illness is a risk for new-onset atrial fibrillation, and patients who previously well controlled are at increased risk of developing rapid ventricular rate (RVR). The primary treatment for rate control in these patients is beta blockers. The prevailing theory is that beta blockers cause melatonin suppression through blockage of sympathetic signaling in the pineal gland. Unfortunately, this class of medication is known to suppress REM sleep, cause nightmares, as well as both sleep onset and sleep maintenance insomnia [36, 37].

The Impact of Poor Sleep on Critical Illness

Delirium

A direct link has not been established between sleep deprivation in the critically ill patients and development of delirium, but severe sleep deprivation and delirium share similar clinical features [38]. Patients in the ICU can develop hypoactive or hyperactive delirium; while both share features of inattentiveness, the treatment and presentation otherwise differ. Hyperactive delirium has features of agitation and restlessness. This form of delirium responds to antipsychotic agents such as seroquel. Hypoactive delirium is often overlooked, as these patients require less staff attention than hyperactive delirium. Hypoactive delirium has features of delayed and blunted responses to stimuli and passive confusion. It does not respond well to pharmacologic intervention.

While the intuitive supposition is that the agitated delirium causes worsening sleep deprivation, and hypoactive delirium is more likely to be a consequence of sleep deprivation, there is no established cause and effect relationship between sleep deprivation and delirium. Both hypoactive and hyperactive delirium are associated with circadian rhythm disturbances; but it is unclear if the circadian disturbance causes the delirium or vice versa [39, 40]. Many medications that cause delirium are also known to cause sleep disturbances, which further supports the concept that severe delirium and sleep disturbances commonly present together [27].

In practice, it is relatively unimportant to establish a cause and effect relationship between delirium and sleep deprivation, as the preventative measures which need to be taken to reduce the rates of delirium have a large overlap with the preventative measures that need to be taken to reduce ICU sleep deprivation. These two issues are heavily intertwined, but encouraging the natural circadian rhythm during the daytime and reducing stimuli at night should help both hypoactive and hyperactive delirium.

Immune System Disturbance

The effect of sleep deprivation on the immune system is complex and incompletely understood. Though intuitively it would seem that a lack of sleep would down regulate the immune response, this appears to be the case mainly in cases with prolonged sleep deprivation (i.e., weeks). Shorter durations of sleep deprivation (2-3 days) do not appear to cause the dysfunction [27].

One study in rats found that after 4 weeks of prolonged sleep deprivation, subjects would develop disseminated infections with opportunistic bacteria [41]. Despite evidence of overwhelming infection seen on post-mortem exam, the rats had leucopenia and did not mount fever responses. On post-mortem exam the rats also had decreased spleen weights, further suggesting immune system failure.

Short-term sleep deprivation has complex effects on the immune system that are not uniform. In healthy human volunteers, after the first 24 hours of sleep deprivation natural killer cell activity is at its nadir [42].

After 48 hours, T-helper cells reach their nadir, but there is a marked increase in natural killer cells, leukocytes and monocytes. Within the first 24 hours of sleep deprivation, there is suppression of some pro-inflammatory cytokines (IL-2), while stimulation of others (ICAM-1, E-selectin, IL-1β, IL-6, TNF-α) is seen [43, 44, 45].

There is very little known on how these effects on the immune system translate into effects on the immune response of critically ill patients. While there are several studies documenting blunted immune response following vaccination in sleep deprived volunteers, [46] this only documents impairment of forming passive immunity and does not translate into interpretations on effects of the immune system responding to infections or other stress states.

Endocrine Dysfunction

The endocrine system is one of the most sensitive to sleep deprivation, even short periods without sleep effects nearly every major endocrine gland. How these hormone changes impact sleep deprived patients, or critically ill patients, is still poorly understood but the widespread deregulation of this regulatory system has been well established.

Sleep deprivation has been linked to decreased insulin secretion, reduced insulin sensitivity, and hyperglycemia [47]. The stress response caused by reduced sleep causes a surge in catecholamines and cortisol [48]. Both the effects on insulin sensitivity and cortisol levels mirror the effects caused by septic shock [49, 50]. This could suggest that these are general stress responses.

TSH, T_3 and T_4 all increase during periods of sleep deprivation [51]. In sick euthyroid syndrome, common in critically ill patients in their early course, all thyroid hormones are decreased [52]. Growth hormone and prolactin levels both are markedly decreased by lack of sleep [51]. This also shows an inverted pattern to patients in septic shock, where both growth hormone and prolactin levels normally increase over the first 24 hours, and then fall below normal levels after several days of sustained illness [53].

Thermoregulation

Naturally people have a regulated temperature cycle that is closely linked to the circadian rhythm. The natural peak body temperature occurs in the late afternoon and will start to wane prior to sleep. During sleep, the body temperature will fall until it reaches a nadir shortly before waking. This drop in temperature can partially be explained by the natural differences in temperatures that occur in the diurnal cycle, but does not directly follow external temperature. One contributing factor to the nightly drop in temperature is due to a loss of shivering during REM sleep, but the drop in temperature starts well prior to REM sleep.

It is not completely understood how temperature affects sleep, but one of the recommendations for all people to optimize sleep hygiene is sleeping in a cool room. This mirrors the natural environment and along with changes in natural sunlight, acts as a signal for the body to promote sleep. Critically ill patients can have their temperature disrupted through a number of mechanisms including fever, cooling and heating blankets, and medications notably paralytics.

While temperature can affect the quality sleep this is not a "one way street"; research has shown that poor sleep quality leads to temperature deregulation as well through disruption of a mechanism called vigilance. Part of the role of human skin is temperature regulation through variations in blood flow in response to external temperatures as well as in response to neurohormonal signaling in response to changes of the core temperature [54]. One study took healthy volunteers who were monitored for 48 hours after normal sleep or a night of sleep deprivation [55]. Over the course of the following two days the patients who were sleep deprived had a significant dissociation of their temperature skin gradients, with increased heat loss in the extremities and increased fluctuations in skin temperature.

Respiratory Dysfunction

Even short periods of sleep deprivation appear to affect a patient's pulmonary mechanics. One study of healthy volunteers after 24 hours of sleep deprivation found that the hypoxic ventilatory response to progressive isocapnic hypoxia was reduced by 29% and that the hypercapnic ventilatory response to a rebreathing technique was reduced by 24% [56]. This is not reflected in changes to PFTs. Another study looking at spirometry of healthy subjects after 30 hours of sleep deprivation found no effect on FEV1 or FVC [57]. This suggests that sleep deprivation mainly causes dysfunction of the respiratory system through the CNS and does not cause significant effects through respiratory fatigue [25].

Post ICU Sleep Disturbances

Post ICU-Syndrome

Post-ICU syndrome is characterized by the development of cognitive, psychiatric or physical disability after treatment in an intensive care setting. Patients are at higher risk if they required mechanical ventilation, but any critically ill patient is at risk of this complication. Post-ICU syndrome is reported to occur in up to 50% of patients who spent more than one week in the ICU, with a frequent complication of cognitive impairment [58]. A study 821 patients in medical and surgical ICUs (where 6% of enrolled patients had prior cognitive impairment) found that 3 months after hospitalization 40% of patients had global cognitive scores at or below 1.5 standard deviations compared to the population mean, which correlates to patients who had moderate TBIs [59]. In the same study 26% of the patients had global cognitive scores at or below 2 standard deviations compared to the population mean, which correlates with mild Alzheimer's disease.

Prevention of post ICU syndrome is an active area of study currently. Minimizing sedation and early mobilization are two things that have shown consistent benefit in reducing the risk of post-ICU syndrome [1]. Optimizing the quality of sleep in critically ill patients has also been suggested as a common sense way to reduce this complication, however there is no evidence yet to support this recommendation.

It is important to screen patients who have recovered from critical illness for development of cognitive impairment, including sleep disturbances. One study of recovered critically ill patients found that 50% of the cohort reported sleep disturbances 1 week after discharge, which would persist for 33% of all patients 6 months after discharge [60].

Identifying patients who are suffering from sleep disturbance and intervening appropriately may help improve physical rehabilitation and mood stabilization. Post-ICU syndrome and post-ICU sleep disturbance are issues which until recently were poorly recognized and where significant progress can be made.

Post-Traumatic Stress Disorder

PTSD caused by critical illness is common and most likely under-diagnosed. One review of 12 studies found that 10-39% of patients treated in the ICU will go on to develop ICU-associated PTSD during their first year after discharge [61]. Risk factors for development of PTSD symptoms after ICU discharge included length of stay, delirium, benzodiazepine use, and if a patient required mechanical ventilation.

One frequent symptom of PTSD is recurrent nightmares, which can lead to somniphobia. PTSD related nightmare disorder is best studied in combat veterans. One of the few medications which has proven effective in that population is prazosin, however it is an off-label use and has not been studied specifically for ICU associated PTSD.

Interventions to Promote Sleep

Sleep disruption in the ICU is a multi-factorial problem; and improving sleep quality for critically ill patients requires a comprehensive approach. The main focus of research has been on impacting the environmental factors of the ICU, especially ambient light and noise, but the success in trials focusing on ICU have been limited. This should not be interpreted to say that reducing light and noise levels cannot have benefit, but instead to say that it is insufficient on its own. An effective model for optimizing sleep quality in the ICU requires a team to tackle all of the issues discussed in this chapter.

A commitment of all the staff needs to be made to batch patient care activities as much as possible, to reduce interruption of sleep. Alarms need to be set at the minimum necessary volume to alert staff, and ambient light needs to be reduced to the minimum levels to still safely allow for patient care. Pain and anxiety need to be addressed, but with the knowledge that overmedication may help induction of sleep but will harm sleep quality.

Despite the fact that light and noise only cause 37% of overnight arousals in the ICU, [5] simple interventions to reduce environmental impact on sleep quality can have significant impacts. One study performed in China in ICU patients who recovering from cardiothoracic surgery found that the use of earplugs and eye masks, along with 30 minutes of relaxing music significantly improved sleep latency, sleep depth, and the frequency of arousals [62].

One of the most important interventions is maintaining wakefulness through the daytime with use of natural light and repeated interaction and stimulation. Families should be encouraged to be as active as possible with their critically ill loved ones during the day, but stimulation and night-time should be kept to a minimum. This can be difficult for family members who cannot visit until later in the day, but nevertheless should be strongly encouraged. Both hyperactive and hypoactive delirium should be treated with conservative measures such as keeping patients awake during the daytime, increasing natural daytime light exposure, providing hearing aids and glasses, and gentle redirection.

Medical sleep aids in the critical care setting have little proven benefit and may cause harm through disruption of normal sleep architecture. In 2018 the Society of Critical Care Medicine updated their clinical practice guidelines for prevention and management of pain, agitation/sedation, delirium, immobility and sleep disruption in adult patients [63]. The SCCM does not recommend for or against melatonin use, and grades the evidence for its use as low in the setting of critical illness. This is based off of three small randomized control trials performed in the ICU setting; none of which showed statistically significant improvements in sleep [64, 65, 66]. The SCCM does not recommend for or against dexmedetomidine use, due to low quality of evidence for its use.

This is based on two small randomized controlled trials which found that dexmedetomidine use decreased stage 1 sleep and increased stage 2 sleep, but had no effect on sleep fragmentation or duration of deep sleep [67, 68]. The SCCM specifically advises against use of hypnotics, benzodiazepines, TCAs, antipsychotics, or propofol as sleep aids in the critically ill [63]. This is because of a lack of evidence of efficacy from clinical trials, concern for disruption of sleep architecture, and concern for safety profiles.

For critically ill patients on ventilators, the Society of Critical Care Medicine recommends that patients be maintained overnight on assist control modes of ventilation. This is because patients maintained on pressure support have been found to have higher rates of central sleep apneas and reduced sleep efficiency and in addition, assist control ventilation is associated with more time in REM sleep [63].

CONCLUSION

Critical illness itself appears to disrupt sleep architecture and quality, which is exacerbated by the chaotic environment of the intensive care unit. Reduction in sleep quality has physiologic impact that may exacerbate illness and impair recovery. Sleep dysfunction in the critically ill remains a new field that is incompletely understood, and optimization of sleep for these patients is an area of active study with a large potential for future benefit.

The physical and mental benefits of good sleep often are undervalued in this population, because the complexity of these patients requires around-the-clock vigilance and intervention, but minimizing rest may come at a large price. Sleep is essential in the regulation and homeostasis of the body's most essential functions: regulation of the immune system, endocrine system, metabolic function and thermoregulation. Disruption of sleep is disruption of health.

Pharmacologic intervention has not proven beneficial to improving sleep quality in the critical care setting, but simple common-sense interventions appear to have large potential benefit. Unfortunately, in the busy and chaotic environment of the ICU, common-sense is often uncommon. Getting buy-in from all staff involved in overnight patient care is essential, and formulating a comprehensive plan tackling a combination of medication awareness and environmental stimulation minimization appears to be the most effective strategy.

Because critical illness itself disrupts sleep, this is not a problem to be solved, but instead one to be minimized. Even after patients have recovered from their illness and have successfully left the hospital they remain at risk for sleep disturbances linked to their illness in the form of post-ICU syndrome and PTSD. It is important to educate providers of this relationship so that patients who have recovered from critical illness can be screened for these problems appropriately.

Sleep is a bedrock for health, and its optimization is a necessary part of optimizing a patient's care.

References

[1] Pisani MA, Friese FS et al. Sleep in the Intensive Care Unit. *Am J Respir Crit Care Med.* 2015;191(7):731-38.

[2] Medrzycka-Dabrowska W, et al. Sleep Deprivation in Intensive Care Unit – Systematic Review. *Open Med.* 2018; 13:384–393.

[3] Knauer MP, Haspel JA, Pisani MA. Sleep loss and circadian rhythm disruption in the Intensive Care Unit. *Clin Chest Med* 2015; 36: 419-429.

[4] Cooper AB, Thornley KS, Young GB, Slutsky AS, Stewart TE, Hanly PJ. Sleep in critically ill patients requiring mechanical ventilation. *Chest.* 2000;117(3):809–818.

[5] Gabor JY, et al. Contribution of the intensive care unit environment to sleep disruption in mechanically ventilated patients and healthy subjects. *Am J Respir Crit Care Med.* 2003;167(5):708-15.

[6] Aurell J, Elmqvist D. Sleep in the surgical intensive care unit: continuous polygraphic recording of sleep in nine patients receiving

postoperative care. *Br Med J (Clin Res Ed).* 1985;290(6474):1029-32.

[7] Freedman NS, Gazendam J, Levan L, et al. Abnormal sleep/wake cycles and the effect of environmental noise on sleep disruption in the intensive care unit. *Am J Respir Crit Care Med* 2001;163: 451–7.

[8] Krueger JM, Majde JA, Rector DM. Cytokines in immune function and sleep regulation. *Handb Clin Neurol*. 2011;98: 229-240.

[9] Krueger JM. The Role of Cytokines in Sleep Regulation. *Current Pharmaceutical Design.* 2008; 14(32):3408-3416(9).

[10] Bihari S, et al. Factors affecting sleep quality of patients in intensive care unit. *J Clin Sleep Med*. 2012 Jun 15;8(3):301-7.

[11] Berglund B, Lindvall T, Schwela DH: *Guidelines for Community Noise Geneva: World Health Organization*; 1999 (http://whqlibdoc.who.int/hq/1999/a68672.pdf).

[12] Information on levels of environmental noise requisite to protect public health and welfare with an adequate margin of safety. *Arlington (VA): Environmental Protection Agency Office of Noise Abatement and Control*; 1974 Mar. Report No.: 550/9-74-004. Accessed on 8/19/2019.

[13] Centers for Disease Control and Prevention. *What noises cause hearing loss?* www.cdc.gov/nceh/hearing_loss/what_noises_cause_hearing_loss.html. Accessed on 8/19/2019.

[14] Darbyshire JL, Young JD. An investigation of sound levels on intensive care units with reference to the WHO guidelines. *Crit Care.* 2013;17(5):R187.

[15] Aaron JN, Carlisle CC, Carskadon MA, et al. Environmental noise as a cause of sleep disruption in an intermediate respiratory care unit. *Sleep* 1996; 19:707–10.

[16] Topf M, Davis JE. Critical care unit noise and rapid eye movement (REM) sleep. *Heart Lung* 1993;22: 252–8.

[17] Nannapaneni S, Lee SJ, et al. Preliminary noise reduction efforts in a medical intensive care unit. *Hospitalist Practice* 2015;43: 94-100.

[18] Tamburri LM, et al. Nocturnal care interactions with patients in critical care units. *Am J Crit Care.* 2004;13(2):102-12.

[19] Meyer TJ, et al. Adverse environmental conditions in the respiratory and medical ICU settings. *Chest* 1994;105:1211–1216.

[20] Weinhouse GL, Schwab RJ. Sleep in the critically ill patient. Sleep 2006;29:707–716.

[21] Freedman NS, Kotzer N, Schwab RJ. Patient perception of sleep quality and etiology of sleep disruption in the intensive care unit. *Am J Respir Crit Care Med* 1999;159:1155–1162.

[22] Simon PM, Zurob AS, Wies WM, Leiter JC, Hubmayr RD. Entrainment of respiration in humans by periodic lung inflations: effect of state and CO(2). *Am J Respir Crit Care Med* 1999;160:950–960.

[23] Parthasarathy S, Tobin MJ. Effect of ventilator mode on sleep quality in critically ill patients. *Am J Respir Crit Care Med.* 2002;166(11): 1423-29.

[24] Beltrami FG, et al. Sleep in the intensive care unit. *J Bras Pneumol.* 2015;41(6):539-46.

[25] Pulak LM, Jensen L. Sleep in the Intensive Care Unit: A Review. *J Intensive Care Med*. 2016;31(1):14-23.

[26] Weinhouse GL. Pharmacology I: effects on sleep of commonly used ICU medications. *Crit Care Clin*. 2008;24(3):477-91.

[27] Kamdar BB, Needham DM, Collop NA. Sleep deprivation in critical illness: its role in physical and psychological recovery. *J Intensive Care Med*. 2012;27(2):97-111.

[28] Murphy PJ. et al. Nonsteroidal anti-inflammatory drugs affect normal sleep patterns in humans. *Physiol Behav*. 1994;55(6):1063-66.

[29] Girard TD. Et al. Haloperidol and Ziprasidone for Treatment of Delirium in Critical Illness. *N Engl J Med* 2018; 379:2506-2516.

[30] Richelson E, Souder T. Binding of antipsychotic drugs to human brain receptors: focus on newer generation antipsychotics. *Life Sci.* 2000;68: 29–39.

[31] Miller DD. Atypical Antipsychotics: Sleep, Sedation, and Efficacy. *Prim Care Companion J Clin Psychiatry*. 2004; 6(suppl 2): 3–7.

[32] Giménez S, Clos S, Romero S, Grasa E, Morte A, Barbanoj MJ. Effects of olanzapine, risperidone and haloperidol on sleep

after a single oral morning dose in healthy volunteers. *Psychopharmacology.* 2007;190(4):507-16.

[33] Schweitzer PK. Drugs That Disturb Sleep and Wakefulness. Kryger MH, Roth T, Dement WC, editors. *Principles and Practice of Sleep Medicine. 5th ed.* St. Louis: Elsevier Saunders; 2011. p. 542-60.

[34] Scarpa M. et al. Sleep disturbances and quality of life in postoperative management after esophagectomy for esophageal cancer. *World Journal of Surgical Oncology* 2014, 12:156.

[35] Bosch NA, Cimini J, Walkey AJ. Atrial Fibrillation in the ICU. *Chest.* 2018;154(6):1424-1434.

[36] Bourne RS, Mills GH. Sleep disruption in critically ill patients: pharmacological considerations. *Anaesthesia* 2004; 59:374–384.

[37] Scheer FA, et. al. Repeated Melatonin Supplementation Improves Sleep in Hypertensive Patients Treated with Beta-Blockers: A Randomized Controlled Trial. *Sleep.* 2012;35(10):1395-402.

[38] Mistraletti G, Carloni E, Cigada M, et al. Sleep and delirium in the Intensive Care Unit. *Minerva Anestesiologica.* 2008;74(6): 329-333.

[39] Miyazaki T, Kuwano H, Kato H, et al. Correlation between serum melatonin circadian rhythm and intensive care unit psychosis after thoracic esophagectomy. *Surgery.* 2003;133(6): 662-668.

[40] Fitzgerald JM, Adamis D, et al. Delirium: A disturbance of circadian integrity. *Med Hypotheses.* 2013;81(4):568-76.

[41] Everson CA. Sustained sleep deprivation impairs host defense. *Am J Physiol.* 1993 Nov;265(5 Pt 2):R1148-54.

[42] Dinges DF, Douglas SD, Zaugg L, et al. Leukocytosis and natural killer cell function parallelneurobehavioral fatigue induced by 64 hours of sleep deprivation. *J Clin Invest.* 1994; 93(5): 1930–1939.

[43] Frey DJ, Fleshner M, Wright KP Jr. The effects of 40 hours of total sleep deprivation on inflammatory markers in healthy young adults. *Brain Behav Immun.* 2007; 21(8):1050–1057.

[44] Irwin M, McClintick J, Costlow C, Fortner M, White J, Gillin JC. Partial night sleep deprivation reduces natural killer and cellular immune responses in humans. *FASEB J.* 1996; 10(5):643–653.

[45] Born J, Lange T, Hansen K, Molle M, Fehm HL. Effects of sleep and circadian rhythm on human circulating immune cells. *J Immunol.* 1997; 158(9):4454–4464.

[46] Spiegel K, Sheridan JF, Van CE. Effect of sleep deprivation on response to immunization. *JAMA.* 2002; 288(12):1471–1472.

[47] Spiegel K, Tasali E, Leproult R, Van Cauter E. Effects of poor and short sleep on glucose metabolism and obesity risk. *Nat Rev Endocrinol.* 2009;5(5):253-261.

[48] Spiegel K, Leproult R, Van Cauter E. Impact of sleep debt on metabolic and endocrine function. *Lancet.* 1999;354(9188):1435-1439.

[49] Van Cromphaut SJ, Vanhorebeek I, Van den Berghe G. Glucose metabolism and insulin resistance in sepsis. *Curr Pharm Des.* 2008;14(19):1887-99.

[50] Vardas K, Apostolou K, Briassouli E, et al., Early Response Roles for Prolactin Cortisol and Circulating and Cellular Levels of Heat Shock Proteins 72 and 90α in Severe Sepsis and SIRS. *Biomed Res Int.* 2014;2014: 803561. doi: 10.1155/2014/803561.

[51] Van Cauter E. Endocrine physiology. In: Kryger M, Roth T, Dement WC, eds. *Principles and Practice of Sleep Medicine*. Philadelphia, PA: Elsevier/Saunders; 2005.

[52] Luo B, Yu Z, Li Y. Thyroid hormone disorders and sepsis. *Biomed Mater Eng.* 2017;28(s1): S237-S241. doi: 10.3233/BME-171646.

[53] Vanhorebeek I, Langouche L, Van den Berghe G. Endocrine aspects of acute and prolonged critical illness. *Nat Clin Pract Endocrinol Metab.* 2006;2(1):20-31.

[54] Romeijn N. et al. Sleep, vigilance, and thermosensitivity. *Eur J Physiol* (2012) 463:169–176.

[55] Romeijn N. et al. Cold hands, warm feet: sleep deprivation disrupts thermoregulation and its association with vigilance. *Sleep.* 2012 Dec 1;35(12):1673-83.

[56] White DP, Douglas NJ, et al. Sleep deprivation and the control of ventilation. *Am Rev Respir Dis.* 1983 Dec;128(6):984-6.

[57] Chen HI, Tang YR. Sleep loss impairs inspiratory muscle endurance. *Am Rev Respir Dis*. 1989;140(4):907-909.

[58] Rawal G, Yadav S, Kumar R. Post-intensive Care Syndrome: an Overview. *J Transl Int Med*. 2017 Jun; 5(2): 90–92.

[59] Pandharipande PP, Girard TD, et al. Long-Term Cognitive Impairment after Critical Illness. *N Engl J Med* 2013; 369:1306-1316.

[60] McKinley S, Aitken LM, et al. Sleep and other factors associated with mental health and psychological distress after intensive care for critical illness. *Intensive Care Med 2012*;38:627–633.

[61] Davydow DS, Gifford JM, Desai SV, Needham DM, Bienvenu OJ. Posttraumatic stress disorder in general intensive care unit survivors: a systematic review. *Gen Hosp Psychiatry*. 2008;30(5):421-434.

[62] Hu RF, Jiang XY, Hegadoren KM, Zhang YH. Effects of earplugs and eye masks combined with relaxing music on sleep, melatonin and cortisol levels in ICU patients: a randomized controlled trial. *Crit Care*. 2015;19: 115.

[63] Devlin JW, et al. Clinical Practice Guidelines for the Prevention and Management of Pain, Agitation/Sedation, Delirium, Immobility, and Sleep Disruption in Adult Patients in the ICU. *Crit Care Med*. 2018 Sep;46(9): e825-e873.

[64] Bourne RS, Mills GH, Minelli C: Melatonin therapy to improve nocturnal sleep in critically ill patients: Encouraging results from a small randomised controlled trial. *Crit Care 2008*; 12:R52.

[65] Shilo L, Dagan Y, Smorjik Y, et al: Effect of melatonin on sleep quality of COPD intensive care patients: A pilot study. *Chronobiol Int* 2000; 17:71–76.

[66] Ibrahim MG, Bellomo R, Hart GK, et al: A double-blind placebocontrolled randomised pilot study of nocturnal melatonin in tracheostomised patients. *Crit Care Resusc* 2006; 8:187–191.

[67] Alexopoulou C, Kondili E, Diamantaki E, et al: Effects of dexmedetomidine on sleep quality in critically ill patients: A pilot study. *Anesthesiology* 2014; 121:801–807.

[68] Nishikimi M, Numaguchi A, Takahashi K, et al: Effect of administration of ramelteon, a melatonin receptor agonist, on duration of stay in the ICU: A single-center, randomized, placebo-controlled trial. *Crit Care Med* 2018; 46:1099–1105.

In: New Research on Sleep …
Editor: Olivier Ratté
ISBN: 978-1-53616-882-2

Chapter 3

SLEEPINESS PERCEPTION AND INSOMNIA IDENTITY: A NETWORK APPROACH

Daniel Ruivo Marques[1,*], Ana Allen Gomes[2], Vanda Clemente[3] and Maria Helena Pinto de Azevedo[4]

[1]Department of Education and Psychology,
University of Aveiro, Aveiro, Portugal
[2]Faculty of Psychology and Educational Sciences,
University of Coimbra, Aveiro, Portugal
[3]Coimbra University Hospital Centre (CHUC),
Sleep Medicine Centre, Coimbra, Portugal
[4]Faculty of Medicine, University of Coimbra,
Coimbra, Portugal

ABSTRACT

Recently, insomnia has been conceptualized as a continuum or dimensional entity comprising four groups: "complaining poor sleepers [CP]," "noncomplaining poor sleepers [NP]," "complaining good sleepers [CG]," and "noncomplaining good sleepers" [NG]. It is well recognized

* Corresponding Author's E-mail: drmarques@ua.pt.

that sleepiness is one of the daytime impairments in insomnia disorder. However, the importance that daytime sleepiness has in insomnia is not clear-cut. In the last years, sleep researchers have proposed a difference between sleepiness propensity and sleepiness perception. In insomnia, researchers and clinicians suggest that sleepiness perception seems to be more relevant than sleepiness propensity. In this line, a brief sleepiness perception measure, the *Daytime Sleepiness Perception Scale* (DSPS-4), which comprises four items, was developed. In the present study, we used network analysis technique to create networks separately for each one of the four "insomnia identity" groups. Data from 673 undergraduate university students were collected. The results showed different network profiles concerning the four sleepiness perception items across the groups. In particular, as to CP group, the most central symptom was item 1 (i.e., During the day, I feel excessively sleepy, full of sleep) in all the centrality measures considered. These findings may help to further understand the role of daytime sleepiness in different insomnia phenotypes and to better target the clinical intervention to the stronger nodes or symptoms.

Keywords: sleepiness, insomnia, insomnia identity, network analysis

INTRODUCTION

Insomnia disorder is defined as the subjective perception of difficulty in falling asleep, difficulty staying sleep, or waking up earlier than the desired time, occuring despite adequate circumstances and opportunity for sleep (AASM, 2014; APA, 2013). These complaints should be necessarily accompanied by daytime impairments (e.g., fatigue, sleepiness, irritability, mood disturbance, cognitive difficulties). Therefore, the "gold standard" for diagnosing insomnia is the clinical interview (Riemann et al., 2017). There is consensus among sleep experts that insomnia, beyond constituting a sleep disorder *per se*, may be considered a pivotal symptom or process in several psychological and physical disorders (transdiagnostic). In this viewpoint, it seems more germane to consider insomnia as a dimension rather than a simple category. In this sense, Lichstein (2017) suggests that it may be useful to consider four groups regarding insomnia – at least in research in this initial stage. The first proposed group, "*complaining poor sleepers* [CP]" is the one, in theory, encompassing the classic insomnia patients; the second group, "*noncomplaining poor sleepers* [NP]," would cover individuals who experience poor sleep but do not self-report insomnia; the third group, "*complaining good sleepers* [CG]," would be constituted by individuals who self-report insomnia complaint but would have good sleep; and, finally, the fourth group, the "*noncomplaining good sleepers*," is the group constituted by the true healthy sleepers [NG] without complaints either of insomnia or poor sleep quality. Thus, two variables are considered to compose this 2 x 2 contingency table: the insomnia complaint (present or absent) and poor sleep complaint (present or absent) (Lichstein, 2017). These groups enable us to outline the importance of insomnia as a subjective complaint/disorder and the relevance that cognitive restructuring techniques may have in insomnia's management, for instance.

Sleepiness is a complex construct within sleep medicine. All over the years, it has been defined as the physiological tendency to fall asleep (i.e., sleep propensity). Notwithstanding, sleepiness seems to be a multidimensional construct (Kim & Young, 2005). One of the principal divisions is between *sleepiness propensity* and *sleepiness perception* (Johns, 2009). Briefly, sleepiness propensity is defined as the unintended propensity for dozing/falling asleep in various everyday situations, whereas sleepiness perception concerns to subjective evaluation of the individual about her/his feeling of sleepiness. In insomnia, sleepiness is among several possible diurnal consequences, however, not all patients complain about it. In the last years, some authors have suggested that sleepiness perception may be a more compromised sleepiness facet rather than propensity (Marques, Gomes, & Azevedo, 2019a). Sleepiness is an important topic in insomnia research (Marques et al., 2019a). In the main official classifications of insomnia, daytime sleepiness is included as one of the criteria to indicate associated daytime impairment (AASM, 2014; APA, 2013). In a recent study, Marques et al. (2019a) reported in detail the psychometric characteristics of the "Daytime Sleepiness Perception Scale" (DSPS-4), a brief instrument to measure daytime sleepiness perception as a complementary measure to the Epworth Sleepiness Scale (ESS) which is the most used sleepiness scale (Johns, 1991, 1992). The authors compared the DSPS-4 items' mean scores of self-reported insomniacs with self-reported non-insomniacs and found that sleepiness perception both in total score and individual items was higher in "insomnia" group, and, in addition, it was observed that the correlation matrix of various psychological and sleep-related measures were stronger for DSPS-4 than for ESS (Marques et al., 2019a). Furthermore, in a subset of participants (first- and second-year students) from the overall sample of the present study, the correlations between DSPS-4 individual items and ESS total score ranged from .23 (item 3: "During the day, I feel that my performance is impaired by being sleepy") to .42 (item 4: "During the day, I feel the need to take a nap"), both p's < 0.001 (Rosmaninho et al., 2010).

The network analysis (NA) constitutes a new alternative to the latent variables paradigm. While latent models posit that manifest or observable indicators are accounted by a non-observable or latent variable, the NA sees the symptoms or observable indicators as causal which, in interaction, originate the clinical disorders, for example (Borsboom, 2017). Put simply, a network is a set of nodes or elements linked by edges or ties. The network analysis enables an interesting visualization of the nodes and edges and gives quantitative indicators of the importance of the nodes which comprise the networks (the so-called "centrality measures"). Moreover, this framework sees the disorders, for example, as systems of mutually reinforcing symptoms and explores the potential of these symptom-symptom interactions (McNally, 2016; Nuijten, Deserno, Cramer, & Borsboom, 2016). The network perspective suggests that disorders emerge as highly connected clusters (i.e., networks) of symptoms, and that these clusters are created by direct interactions between symptoms.

The network approach has been applied recently in psychopathology and behavioral sciences (Borsboom, 2017). To our knowledge, only two publications relate sleep/insomnia to the network approach. One is an empirical paper on the relationship between insomnia severity and personality (Dekker, Blanken, & Van Someren, 2017) and the other is an editorial inciting researchers to use network analyses within sleep medicine field in the future (Marques & Azevedo, 2018).

Considering this background, the aim of this exploratory study was two-fold: (1) to replicate the sleep types of CP, NP, CG and NG in a homogenous sample of young-adults given that there are age-related differences in the self-reported pattern of sleep difficulties (Azevedo et al., 2007; Roth et al., 2006) and in the internal metrics used to assess sleep quality (Zilli, Ficca, & Salzarulo, 2009); and (2) to examine the sleepiness perception profile within the four groups using NA.

METHODS

Participants

In this study, data from 673 undergraduates (n = 441; 65.5% females), all single, from a public Portuguese university were analysed. An initial pool of 713 responses were collected but for the principal aims of the present study, we only considered cases with no missing values (94.4%) in insomnia and sleep quality questions (cf. Measures section). Mean age for both the total (n = 713) and selected samples (n = 673) were identical: M = 19.2; SD = 1.25; Min = 17; Max = 24.

In Table 1, it is displayed an overall characterization of the total sample with regard to perceived physical and mental health, body mass index (BMI), snoring, insomnia, and subjective sleep quality.

Most students had "very good/good" physical health (83.6%) and mental health (77.3%). Total sample BMI mean score was 21.2 (SD = 2.54); 9.8% participants were underweight (BMI < 18.5), 80.9% normal weight (BMI 18.5-24.9) and 6.6% overweight/obese (BMI ≥ 25). For the current study, this measure is very important given its association with sleepiness propensity as observed in several studies (Marques et al., 2019a). Snoring was reported "never/rarely" by 76%. 10.2% of the students reported insomnia "quite often/almost always."

Of the total sample, 55.7% of the participants classified their subjective sleep quality as "very good/good."

Table 1. Overall characteristics of total sample (*N* = 713)

	n (%)
Perceived physical health	
Good/Very good	596 (83.6%)
Neither good/Poor	93 (13%)
Very poor/Poor	18 (2.5%)
Missing	6 (0.8%)
Perceived mental health	
Good/Very good	551 (77.3%)
Neither good/Poor	125 (17.5%)
Very poor/Poor	30 (4.2%)
Missing	7 (1%)
BMI (kg/m^2)	
Underweight (BMI < 18.5)	70 (9.8%)
Normal weight (BMI 18.5-24.9	577 (80.9%)
Overweight (BMI 25.0-29.9)	42 (5.9%)
Obese (BMI ≥ 30)	5 (0.7%)
Missing	19 (2.7%)
Snoring	
Never/Rarely	542 (76%)
Often	33 (4.6%)
Almost always/Always	15 (2.1%)
Do not know	113 (15.8%)
Missing	10 (1.4%)
Insomnia	
Almost never	397 (55.7%)
Quite seldom	209 (29.3%)
Quite often	62 (8.7%)
Almost always	11 (1.5%)
Missing	34 (4.8%)
Subjective sleep quality	
Very good/good	472 (66.2%)
Satisfactory	199 (27.9%)
Poor/very poor	36 (5.0%)
Missing	397 (0.8%)

Measures

The following self-reported measures were used:

Subjective sleep quality. Sleep quality was evaluated recurring to the question "Ever since you can remember, how has your sleep quality been?." This variable was dichotomized into two categories: "good sleepers" (i.e., very good, good, and satisfactory) and "poor sleepers" (i.e., poor and very poor) (Marques, Gomes, Ferreira, & Azevedo, 2016);

Self-reported insomnia. To measure self-reported insomnia, we used the item 12 of the Eysenck Personality Inventory: "I suffer from insomnia" (EPI-12, Eysenck & Eysenck, 1964). The item is scored 1 = "almost never," 2 = "quite seldom," 3 = "quite often," and 4 = "almost always." Responses were dichotomized to indicate the presence ("quite often" and "almost always") or absence ("almost never," and "quite seldom") of insomnia.

Daytime Sleepiness Perception Scale (DSPS-4). The DSPS-4 comprises 4 items intended to evaluate subjective perception of sleepiness. The response options are: 0 = never; 1 = rarely; 2 = often; 3 = almost always; 4=always. The sum of the four items originates a composite score which indicates the overall subjective sleepiness perception. No specific time frame is specified in the instructions. In the current study, the Cronbach's alpha considering total sample was .71.

Snoring. Snoring was assessed through the question "I snore during sleep" with response categories of "never, rarely, often, almost always, always, and unknown." This variable is included due to its relevance in sleepiness studies (Marques et al., 2019a).

Body Mass Index (BMI). Self-reported current body weight and height was used to calculate BMI (kg/m^2).

Self-Perceived Health. Self-perceived physical and mental health status was assessed with two questions: "Generally, what has your physical health been like?" and "Generally, what has your mental health been like?." Responses options are: very poor (coded as "1"), poor, neither good nor poor, good, and very good (coded as "5").

Procedure

After professors' permission, the set of questionnaires were administered to the students at the beginning/ending of a class session (out of the evaluation period). The researchers ensured the voluntary collaboration and confidentiality of the data. All students returned the questionnaires. Ethical approval for the study was obtained from the last author's Faculty Scientific Council and Ethics Committee. It should be noted that the data used for the current study is based on a previously collected database, which has been used for several publications.

Data Analysis

Descriptive statistics such as frequencies, means and standard deviations were calculated to characterize the sample. Chi-Square test (Fisher's Exact Test) was used to evaluate an eventual association between nominal variables. Cramer's *V* and *Odds Ratio* (OR) were used as effect size measures (Field, 2013). One-way ANOVAs were computed to compare groups and Eta Squared was used as effect measure. Bonferroni corrections to control for type I errors were used for pairwise comparisons. The significance level was set at $p \leq .05$. All these calculations were performed with *IBM SPSS Statistics*, version 25.0.

The network analysis were performed using the JASP software - version 0.9.1 (JASP Team, 2018). The EBICglasso (Extended Bayesian Information criterion) was the used estimator. Centrality measures were calculated to identify nodes that may have a particular importance in the networks. The common centrality indicators are *strength/degree*, *closeness*, and *betweenness*. Overall, higher values of centrality indicators suggest greater importance of the node to the network. *Strength* (or degree) reflect the quantity and the weight of correlations; *closeness* refers to the distance that a particular node has from the remaining nodes, thus, an important node is close to many other nodes of the network, and finally, *betweenness* reflects the number of times a node appears on the shortest path between two other nodes. It was used the Fruchterman-Reingold algorithm to position the more central nodes at the centre of the graphs (Fruchterman & Reingold, 1991). In our NA, DSPS-4 items are represented as nodes and associations among nodes (edges) are displayed as lines which may be more or less thick (according to the weight of the correlation) and blue or red (if the association is positive or negative, respectively).

RESULTS

Contingency Table Analysis

In terms of sleep type's distribution, the results are displayed in Table 2. The NG group constituted the majority of the sample (n = 584, 86.8%) whereas the CP (n = 17, 2.5%) and NP (n = 17, 2.5%) groups were the ones with less sample size (both comprising 17 participants). The CG group distribution was n = 55 (8.2%). Regarding inferential statistics, the results were: Fisher's Exact Test [$p < .001$]; Cramer's $V = 0.293$; $p < .001$; OR = 10.65. Overall, the odds of having an insomnia complaint and poor sleep was 10 greater compared to individuals who have not insomnia complaint.

Table 2. Distribution of sleep types in young-adults sample. The off diagonal groups (boldface numbers) represent the uncoupled sleepers

		Insomnia Complaint	
		Present	Absent
Poor Sleep	Present	17 [CP]	17 [NP]
	Absent	55 [CG]	584 [NG]

Note: CP = complaining poor sleepers; NP = noncomplaining poor sleepers; CG = complaining good sleepers; NG = noncomplaining good sleepers.

Table 3. Mean differences pertaining to sleepiness perception

	CP (n = 17)	NP (n = 17)	CG (n = 55)	NG (n = 584)		Test		Effect Size
	M (SD)	M (SD)	M (SD)	M (SD)	df	F/Welch	p	η^2
During the day, I feel excessively sleepy, full of sleep	1.76 (0.75)	1.88 (0.85)	1.67 (0.74)	1.34 (0.54)	3,36.048	6.955[a]	.001	.053
Being sleepy during the day is a problem for me	1.71 (0.77)	1.94 (0.82)	1.56 (0.71)	1.23 (0.64)	3,662	12.455	<.001	.053
During the day, I feel that my performance is impaired by being sleepy	1.76 (0.90)	2.00 (0.93)	1.69 (0.74)	1.44 (0.71)	3,36.531	4.215[a]	<.001	.026
During the day, I feel the need to take a nap	1.35 (0.86)	1.59 (0.87)	1.22 (0.97)	1.14 (0.80)	3,667	2.088	.101	.009

Note: CP = complaining poor sleepers; NP = noncomplaining poor sleepers; CG = complaining good sleepers; NG = noncomplaining good sleepers.

Bonferroni corrections were applied to correct multiple comparisons. The p-value considered statistically significant was set to .012 (.05/4).

[a]The Welch test (Asymptotically F distributed) was used since the homogeneity of variances was not verified.

Descriptive Statistics

Concerning descriptive statistics, it was observed that in all the DSPS-4 items the CP and NP groups endorsed higher scores compared to CG and NG groups (cf. Table 3). The only exception was for item 4 ("During the day, I feel the need to take a nap").

Network Analysis

After the performance of network analysis for the four insomnia identity groups, it was observed that the association pattern was distinctive for each one of the groups (see Figure 1).

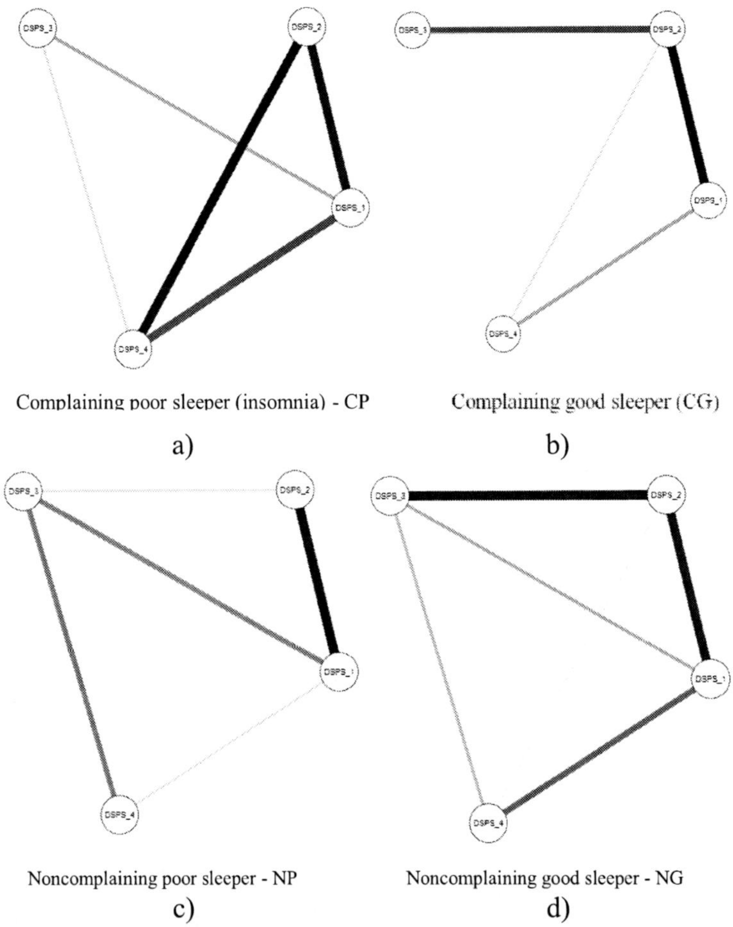

Note: DSPS-1 = During the day, I feel excessively sleepy, full of sleep; DSPS-2 = Being sleepy during the day is a problem for me; DSPS-3 = During the day, I feel that my performance is impaired by being sleepy; DSPS-4 = During the day, I feel the need to take a nap.

Figure 1. Concentration network for insomnia identity groups. Blue lines denote positive associations. Thicker lines represent stronger relationships.

Specifically, in terms of visual analysis, it is evident that in all groups except CP, only positive associations were observed. As to CP, which is the group corresponding to traditional "insomnia," one negative association displayed in red color is visible between item 1 ("During the day, I feel excessively sleepy, full of sleep") and item 4 ("During the day, I feel the need to take a nap") (see Figure 1a).

Moreover, it was observed that item 2 "Being sleepy during the day is a problem for me" and item 3 "During the day, I feel that my performance is impaired by being sleepy" are not associated in both poor sleepers groups (cf. Figures 1a and 1c). In addition, it was observed that item 3 and item 4 items are not associated in both complaining groups (cf. Figures 1a) and 1b).

In order to identify the most important nodes to the networks pertaining to the groups, the centrality measures – *betweenness*, *closeness* and *degree/strength*, were calculated (see Figure 2). We found that in CP group, the most central symptom across the three measures was item 1 (i.e., During the day, I feel excessively sleepy, full of sleep). Concerning NG and CG groups, items 1 and 2 achieved the better centrality results. Regarding NP group, items 1 and 3 were the most important nodes.

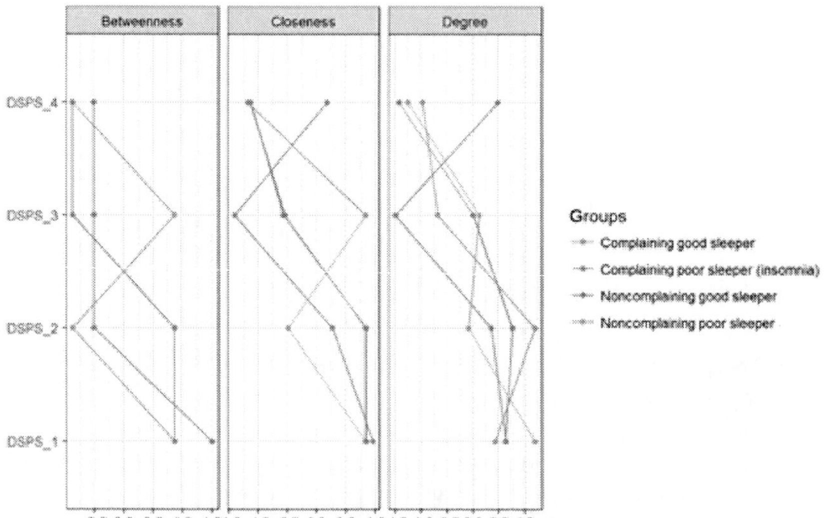

Note: DSPS-1 = During the day, I feel excessively sleepy, full of sleep; DSPS-2 = Being sleepy during the day is a problem for me; DSPS-3 = During the day, I feel that my performance is impaired by being sleepy; DSPS-4 = During the day, I feel the need to take a nap.

Figure 2. Centrality indices (*z*-scores) of the DSPS-4 nodes.

Despite the low sample size of some of the groups, we performed stability and accuracy analyses recurring to nonparametric bootstrapping as an additional analysis. Therefore, edge stability (cf. Figure 3) and centrality stability (cf. Figure 4) were calculated. The number of bootstraps initially executed were 10 and posteriorly 1000 (Epskamp, Borsboom, & Fried, 2018).

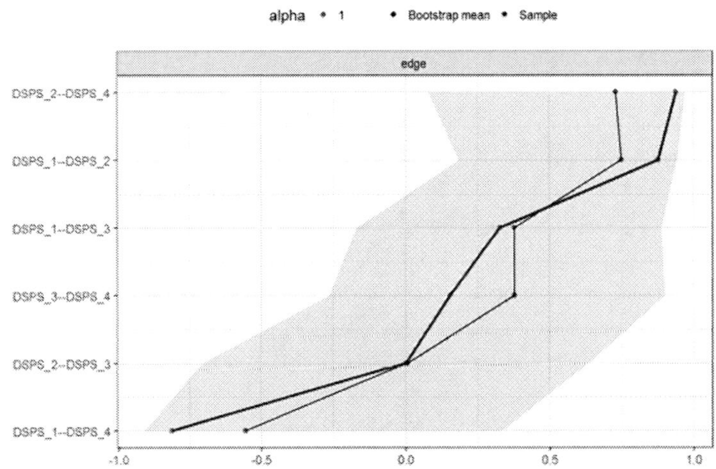

a) Complaining poor sleeper (insomnia)

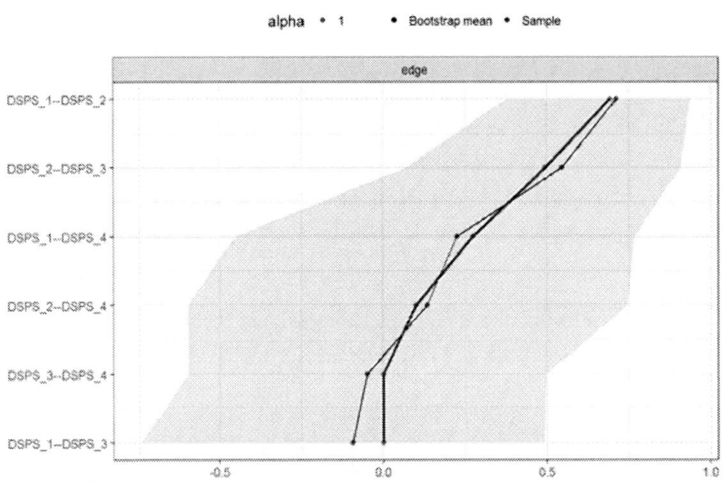

b) Complaining good sleeper

Figure 3. (Continued)

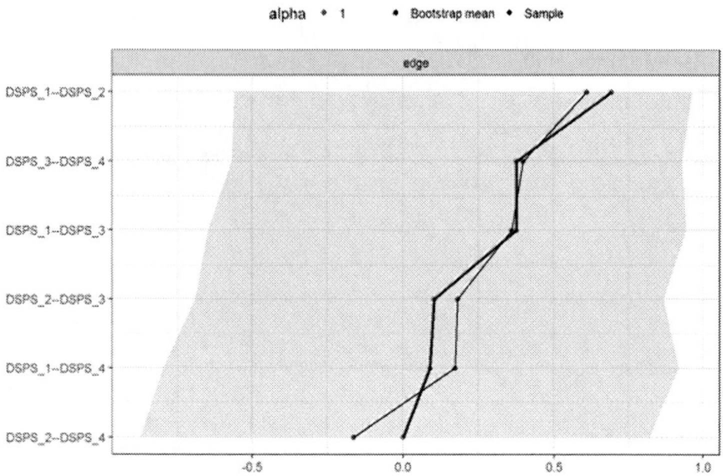

c) Noncomplaining poor sleeper

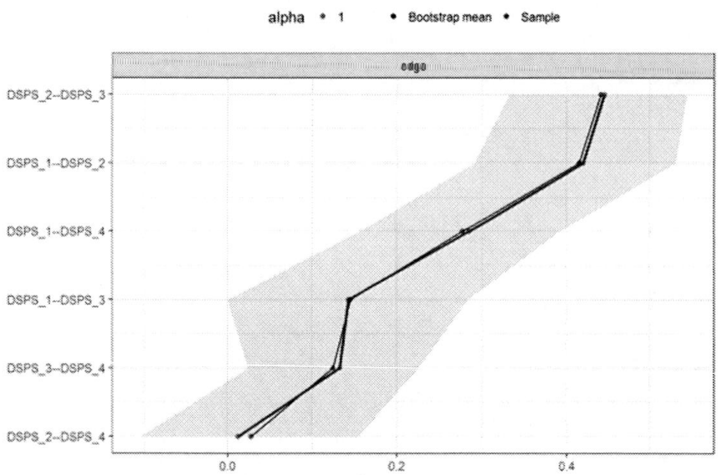

d) Noncomplaining good sleeper

Note: DSPS-1 = During the day, I feel excessively sleepy, full of sleep; DSPS-2 = Being sleepy during the day is a problem for me; DSPS-3 = During the day, I feel that my performance is impaired by being sleepy; DSPS-4 = During the day, I feel the need to take a nap.

Figure 3. Edge stability of the insomnia identity groups.

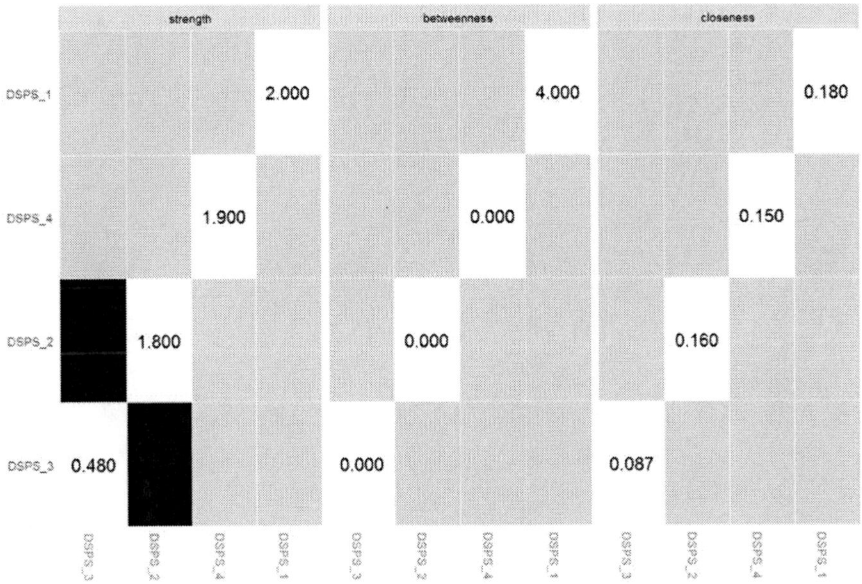

a) Complaining poor sleeper (insomnia)

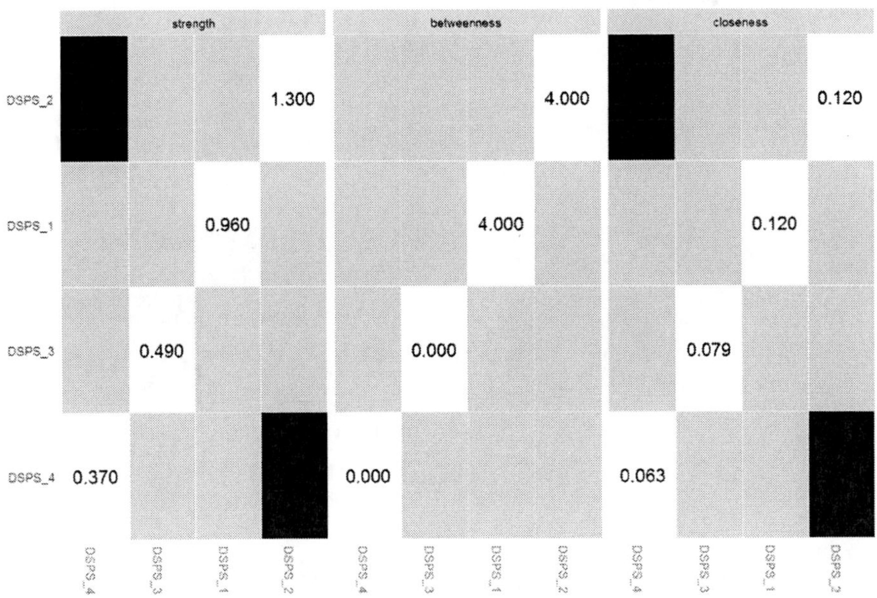

b) Complaining good sleeper

Figure 4 (Continued)

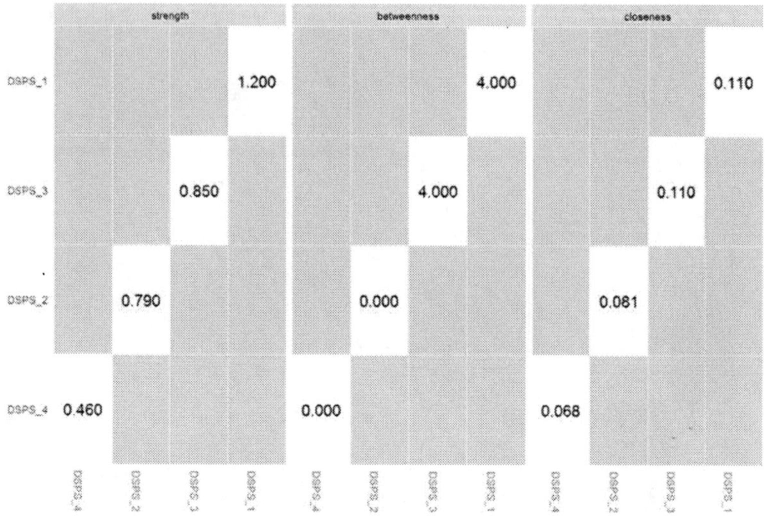

c) Noncomplaining poor sleeper

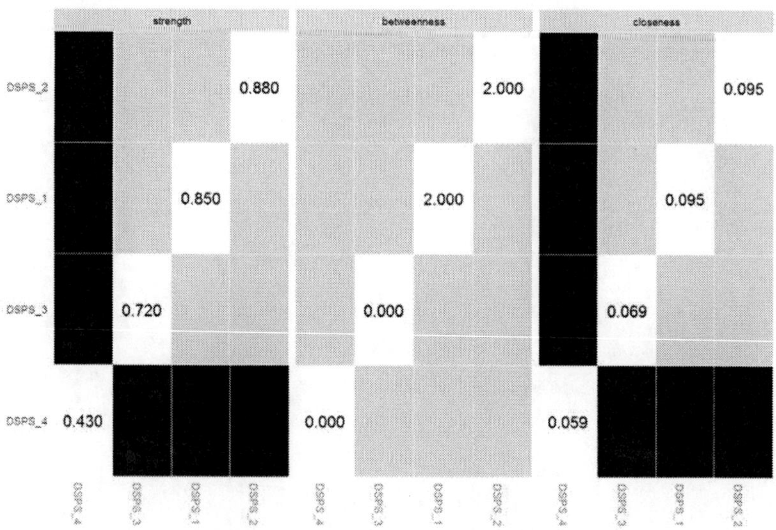

d) Noncomplaining good sleeper

Note: DSPS-1 = During the day, I feel excessively sleepy, full of sleep; DSPS-2 = Being sleepy during the day is a problem for me; DSPS-3 = During the day, I feel that my performance is impaired by being sleepy; DSPS-4 = During the day, I feel the need to take a nap.

Figure 4. Centrality stability of the insomnia identity groups.

DISCUSSION

Most of the participants in this study reported very good/good physical (83.6%) and mental health (77.3%); the majority had a normal weight and 76% "never/rarely" snored. Of the total sample, subjective sleep quality was considered "very good/good" by 55.7%, "satisfactory" by 27.9% and 10% of the students reported insomnia.

In this report, we aimed to examine the sleep type's distribution of CP, NP, CG, and NG and daytime sleepiness perception indicators across the same groups in a sample of young adults.

Concerning to sleep types, the great majority of participants are included in NG group (86.8%); the CG group comprises 8.2%; and both CP and NP represent 2.5%, respectively, whereas in the Lichstein's study (2017) the percentages are 55%, 10%, 19%, and 16%, respectively.

Methodological differences such as sample characteristics and measures used for assessing sleep parameters may account for discrepancies between the two studies. However, it worth noting that CG percentage in both studies are similar.

As to sleepiness perception individual differences in mean scores across the four groups, we find that NP and CP levels of sleepiness are significantly higher compared to remaining groups, with the exception of item 4 whose difference does not achieve statistical significance albeit the same tendency is observable.

Regarding the NA results, it is observed differential network patterns. Unfortunately, as no other study investigated subjective sleepiness perception, it is impossible to compare our results.

Overall, "complaining" groups individuals' do not manifest an association between items 3 ("During the day, I feel that my performance is impaired by being sleepy") and 4 ("During the day, I feel the need to take a nap"). On the other hand, "poor sleepers" do not manifest association between items 2 ("Being sleepy during the day is a problem for me") and 3 ("During the day, I feel that my performance is impaired by being sleepy"). Besides, it is evident that item 4 presents the lower centrality measures compared to the other three items of DSPS-4 suggesting that the latter may be a less relevant item for evaluating sleepinees perception. One interesting point to explore in future research is whether this item constitutes a "transition/bridge" node between sleepiness perception and sleepiness propensity.

These findings seem to be in line with the Alapin's et al. (2000) claim that daytime symptoms do not reflect a unitary construct among insomnia individuals.

A main finding of the current study is the observed negative association only between item 1 and item 4 in CP. Despite previous studies have shown that the four DSPS-4 items are correlated and account for a single factor entitled sleepiness perception (Marques et al., 2019a), it seems that item 4 is more sleepiness propensity-related (Rosmaninho et al., 2010) and individuals with insomnia disorder may have a lower sleep propensity (APA, 2013).

Despite the interesting results obtained in this exploratory study, some limitations should be outlined. The insomnia "status" was defined based on a single item drawn from EPI, which is a personality measure; the sleep-related indicators were all based on subjective/self-report measures. One should note that perhaps the major limitation of this study is the small sample size of some groups, particularly, the CP and the NP (both groups have n = 17). Nonetheless, the patterns seem to be robust (even when we consider the bootstrapping analyses). However, these results should be seen as a first attempt to the topic and replication with more balanced groups are needed.

This is a study comprising a non-clinical sample and therefore generalization to well-defined clinical groups should be made carefully. However, if we consider insomnia as a dimensional entity whose understanding can benefit from studies with community samples, then these kind of researches as ours may reveal important apects for clinical practice (Marques, Gomes, & Azevedo, 2019b).

Future studies should investigate the distribution of these quadrants among other groups either clinical or nonclinical. Besides, it would be important to use standardized measures for measuring insomnia and poor sleep in order to compare the groups in a cross-cultural way.

In summarizing, the current study adds to the literature that the four groups proposed by Lichstein (2017) are present in a nonclinical sample constituted by young adults, specifically, undergraduate students. Based on the psychological and sleep-derived measures, the uncoupled sleepers constitute individuals who deserve in-depth studies in order to understand better the insomnia developmental pathway.

ACKNOWLEDGMENTS

The authors would like to express their gratitude to the professors and undergraduates who participated in this research.

REFERENCES

Alapin, I., Fichten, C., Libman, E., Creti, L., Bailes, S., & Wright, J. (2000). How is good and poor sleep in older adults and college students related to daytime sleepiness, fatigue, and ability to concentrate? *Journal of Psychosomatic Research*, 49(5), 381-390. doi: 10.1016/S0022-3999(00)00194-X.

American Academy of Sleep Medicine. (2014). *International classification of sleep disorders: Diagnostic and coding manual* (3rd ed.) Westchester.

American Psychiatric Association. (2013). *Diagnostic and statistical manual of mental disorders-5* (5th ed.). Washington, DC: American Psychiatric Association.

Azevedo, M., Soares, M. J., Bos, S., Gomes, A., Maia, B., … Macedo, A. (2009). Perfectionism and sleep disturbance. *World Journal of Biological Psychiatry*, 10(3), 225-233. doi:10.1080/ 15622970701367930.

Borsboom, D. (2017). A network theory of mental disorders. *World Psychiatry*, 16(1), 5-13. doi:10.1002/wps.20375.

Cluydts, R., De Valck, E., Verstraeten, E., & Theys, P. (2002). Daytime sleepiness and its evaluation. *Sleep Medicine Reviews*, 6(2), 83-96. doi:10.1053/smrv.2002.0191.

Dekker, K., Blanken, T., & Van Someren, E. (2017). Insomnia and personality: A network approach. *Brain Sciences*, 7(3), 28. doi:10.3390/brainsci7030028.

Epskamp, S., Borsboom, D., & Fried, E. (2018). Estimating psychological networks and their accuracy: A tutorial paper. *Behavior Research Methods*, 50(1), 195-212. doi:10.3758/s13428-017-0862-1.

Field, A. (2013). *Discovering Statistics using IBM SPSS Statistics* (4th ed.). London: Sage Publications.

Fruchterman, T., & Reingold, E. (1991). Graph drawing by force-directed placement. *Software: Practice and Experience*, 21(1), 1129-1164. doi:10.1002/spe.4380211102.

Johns, M. W. (1991). A new method for measuring daytime sleepiness: The Epworth sleepiness scale. *Sleep*, 16(4), 540-545.

Johns, M. W. (1992). Reliability and factor analysis of the Epworth Sleepiness Scale. *Sleep*, 15(4), 376-381.

Johns, M. (2009). What is excessive daytime sleepiness? In: P. Fulke & S. Vaughan (Eds.), *Sleep deprivation: Causes, effects and treatment* (pp. 59-94). New York: Nova Science Publishers, Inc.

JASP Team (2018). *JASP (Version 0.9.1)* [Computer software].

Kim, H., & Young, T. (2005). Subjective daytime sleepiness: Dimensions and correlates in the general population. *Sleep*, 28, 625-634.

Lichstein, K. (2017). Insomnia identity. *Behaviour Research and Therapy*, 97, 230-241. doi:10.1016/j.brat.2017.08.005.

Marques, D., & Azevedo, M. H. (2018). Potentialities of network analysis for sleep medicine. *Journal of Psychosomatic Research*, 111, 89-90. doi:10.1016/j.jpsychores.2018.05.019.

Marques, D., Gomes, A., & Azevedo, M. H. (2019a). DSPS-4: A brief measure of perceived daytime sleepiness. *Current Psychology*, 38(2), 579-588. doi:10.1007/s12144-017-9638-0.

Marques, D., Gomes, A., & Azevedo, M. H. (2019b). *Utility of studies in community-based populations*. Manuscript submitted for publication.

Marques, D., Gomes, A., Ferreira, M., & Azevedo, M. H. (2016). Don't worry, Sleep well: Predictors of sleep loss over worry. *Sleep and Biological Rhythms*, 14(3), 309-318. doi:10.1007/s41105-016-0060-z.

McNally, R. (2016). Can network analysis transform psychopathology? *Behaviour Research & Therapy*, 86, 95-104. doi:10.1016/j.brat.2016.06.006.

Nuijten, M., Deserno, M., Cramer, A., & Borsboom, D. (2016). Mental disorders as complex networks: An introduction and overview of a network approach to psychopathology. *Clinical Neuropsychiatry*, 13(4-5), 68-76.

Riemann, D., Baglioni, C., Bassetti, C., Bjorvatn, B., Dolenc Groselj, L., Ellis, J., ... Spiegelhalder, K. (2017). European guideline for the diagnosis and treatment of insomnia. *Journal of Sleep Research*, 26(6), 675-700. doi:10.1111/jsr.12594.

Rosmaninho, J., Lopes, M., Quintal, J., Soares, M. J., Maia, B., … Azevedo, M. H. (2010). Daytime sleepiness in medical students. *Journal of Sleep Research*, 19 (suppl. 2), 178.

Roth, T., Jaeger, S., Jin, R., Kalsekar, A., Stang, P., & Kessler, R. (2006). Sleep problems, comorbid mental disorders, and role functioning in the national comorbidity survey replication. *Biological Psychiatry*, 60(12), 1364-1371. doi:10.1016/j.biopsych.2006.05.039.

Zilli, I., Ficca, G., & Salzarulo, P. (2009). Factors involved in sleep satisfaction in the elderly. *Sleep Medicine*, 10(2), 233-239. doi:10.1016/j.sleep.2008.01.004.

In: New Research on Sleep …
Editor: Olivier Ratté
ISBN: 978-1-53616-882-2

Chapter 4

THE MULTIPLE SLEEP LATENCY TEST (MSLT) IN NARCOLEPSY-1

J. J. Ortega-Albás, MD, R. López García, MD, M. Badenes Lengua, MD, S. Carratalá Monfort, MD, A. Martínez Martínez, MD and P. Ortega, MD
Sleep Unit. Universitary General Hospital of Castellón.
Castellón de la Plana, Spain

ABSTRACT

Multiple Sleep Latency Test (MSLT) is the standard physiological measure of sleepiness.

It conceptualizes sleepiness as the tendency to fall asleep by measuring the speed of falling asleep. Also MSLT has gained acceptance within the field of sleep as standard method of quantifying sleepiness.

In the spring of 1976, Mary Carskadon and colleagues established protocol and development of the MSLT. This test was then formally applied to the clinical evaluation of sleepiness in patients with narcolepsy and later, in patient with OSAS.

We present results in MSLT of forty patients diagnosed of narcolepsy-1 and review the actual protocol.

INTRODUCTION

The identification and characterization of excessive daytime sleepiness (EDS) is one of the fundamental tasks of sleep specialists. It is defined as drowsiness that occurs in situations in which the individual should be awake and alert [1].

Pathological somnolence occurs in association with disorders and conditions such as narcolepsy, hypersomnia and sleep deprivation.

The first International Congress on Narcolepsy [2] held in 1975 mapped clinical neurophysiological tests that should be used for its diagnosis. The school of Standford was in charge of its development. First, they created the polisomnogram (PSG) to monitor bioelectric brain activity and vital functions during sleep and defined the multiple sleep latency test (MSLT).

Richardson [3] and Mitler [4], from Mary Carskadon´s group observed that subjects with Narcolepsy-Cataplexy had a short sleep latency and an abnormal distribution of stages and states during the onset of nocturnal sleep, as well as at the begining of sleep during daytime naps, with frequent occurence of early REM sleep.

A year earlier Carskadon [5] suggested that sleep latency in programmed and controlled naps should provide a useful tool in the evaluation of pathological sleepiness. In turn, she defined sleep latency as the time that elapses from the moment an individual tries to sleep until EEG sleep pattern arise.

The main lines of the usefulness of MSLT in somnolgy were outlined: the objective evaluation of sleepiness and the diagnosis of narcolepsy and other hipersomnias of central origin which have been unchanged.

Basically, the MSLT consist in offering the subject the possibility of sleeping 4-5 naps the morning after a polysomnographic study (PSG), at intervals of 2 hours, to measure the sleep latency and the purpose of REM sleep.

The MSLT has therefore two aspects and two different protocols of action:

A. *Experimental MSLT:* Established for the documentation and quantification of somnolence in the context of sleep deprivation. The patient under study is awakened immediately after sleep arise in any nap.
B. *Clinical MSLT:* The record is prolonged 15 minutes after the beginning of sleep during the naps. The aim is to increase the possibility of REM sleep appearing during nap logs (Sleep Onset REM period or SOREMP).

According to the international classification of sleep disorders we can find different types of central disorders with hypersomnolence.

The main types that will be developed are:

- Narcolepsy type I.
- Narcolepsy type II.
- Idiopatic hypersomnia.

The following entities within this group would also be collected according to the classification:

- Kleine-Levin syndrome.
- Hipersomnia due to medical disorders.
- Hipersomnia due to substances or medications.
- Hipersomnia related to other mental disorders.
- Insuficient sleep syndrome.

Narcolepsy type I (also called Narcolepsy with cataplexy or Gelineau Syndrome is mainly characterized by:

1. Excessive daytime sleepiness and episodes of cataplexy.
2. Brief and refreshing sleep attacks, followed in a few hours of drowsiness.

The episodes of cataplexy, unequal sudden loss of muscle tone, are usually triggered by positive emotional experiences such as laughter (the most frequent), euphoria or surprise and negative one such as crying.

Clinically these attacks involves principally proximal musculature, mainly the lower extremities and the facial musculature, with bilateral ptosis, mandibular dislocation, weakness of the facial muscles ("cataplectic facies").

Patients may be experienced chin tremors, with difficulty in articulating words and abolishing osteotendinous reflexes.

Patients can also refer:

3. Episodes of sleep paralysis.
4. Hypnagogic hallucinations (waking-dream transition) or hypnopompic (dream- waking transition), including visual, auditory and/or tactile phenomena.
5. Automatic behavior during sleep.
6. Fragmented sleep (they have no difficulty for the onset of sleep but for maintenance) with numerous awakenings, which can further aggravate daytime sleepiness.

The International Classification of Sleep Disorders (ICSD-3) [6] includes the following diagnostic criteria for Narcolepsy Type 1 (NT1):

A. The patient has daily periods of irresistible sleep attacks or daytime sleep lapses that occur for at least 3 months.
B. The presence of one or more of the following symptoms:
    1. Cataplexy and average sleep latency equal to or less than 8 minutes and two or more SOREMPs in an MSLT developed in accordance with standard techniques. A SOREMP (within 15 minutes from the start of sleep) in the nocturnal polysomnogram can replace one of the SOREMPs in the MSLT.
    2. Concentration of hypocretin-1 in CSF, (measured by immunoreactivity) less than 110 pg/mL absolute, or <1/3 of

the average values obtained from normal subjects with the same standardized technique. Both criteria A and B must be met.

ICSD-3 suggests repeating the MSLT if NT1 is strongly suspected, but criterion B1 of the TLMS is not met.

The MSLT is therefore a fundamental pillar for the diagnosis of NT1, with a sensitivity of 92.9% and a specificity of 98.6% [7]. Unlike the ICSD-2 version, the last one includes a SOREMP in the previous nocturnal PSG in the total number of SOREMPs needed for the diagnosis of NT1. Although the observation of a nocturnal SOREMP is highly specific for Narcolepsy (99%), the implemented research suggests that adding this period to the total number of SOREMPs does not lead to a significant change in diagnosis [8, 9].

Type II narcolepsy or narcolepsy without cataplexy is similar in most clinical aspects to type I narcolepsy except for the absence, at the time of diagnosis, of apparent episodes of cataplexy. This means that the diagnosis could change in patients who develop episodes of cataplexy during the course of the disease. One of the differences from type I narcolepsy is observed in the levels of hypocretin-1 in the (CSF) which are usually normal among patients who have narcolepsy without cataplexy, while in those who have type I narcolepsy they are <110 pg/mL or undetectable.

According to the diagnostic criteria (ICSD-3) [6], the following items must be met:

A. The patient has daily periods of irresistible sleep attacks or daytime sleep lapses that occur for at least 3 months.
B. An average sleep latency ≤ 8 minutes and 2 or more SOREMPs in the MSLT.
C. SOREMP (within 15 minutes of sleep onset) in the preceding PSG can replace one of the SOREMPs in the MSLT.
D. Absence of cataplexy.

E. Concentration of hypocretin-1 n measured at > 110 pg/mL or > 1/3 of the average values obtained from normal subjects with the same technique. The hypersomnolence and/or MSLT found cannot be explained by other causes such as insufficient sleep, obstructive apnea, delay phase disorder or the effect of medication or withdrawal of substances.

Idiopathic hypersomnia is characterized by excessive daytime sleepiness despite a longer than average duration of nighttime sleep. Patients report a feeling of dullness or confusion in the morning. Daytime naps are long and not refreshing compared to those of narcoleptic patients.

The criteria included in (ICSD-3) [6] for idiopatic hypersomnia are the following:

A. The patient has daily periods of irresistible sleep attacks or daytime sleep lapses that occur for at least 3 months.
B. Absence of cataplexy.
C. An MSLT shows less than 2 SOREMPs or none during the latency test if the REM latency in the previous PSG was less than or equal to 15 minutes.
D. The presence of at least one of the following:
    1. The MSLT shows an average sleep latency ≤ 8 minutes.
    2. The total sleep time of 24 hours is ≥ 660 minutes (usually 12 to 14 hours) PSG performed after the correction of lack of sleep, or by wrist actigraphy in association with a daily sleep (for at least seven days).
E. Insufficient sleep syndrome has been ruled out (bed time demonstrated with at least one week of actigraphy).
F. The hypersomnolence and/or MSLT found cannot be explained by other causes such as insufficient sleep, obstructive apnea, delay phase disorder or the effect of medication or withdrawal of substances.

Table 1. Relationship between the different types of hypersomnia and the diagnostic criteria (clinical, MSLT, hypocretin and HLA)

ICSD-3 TYPES	DIAGNOSTIC CRITERIA
Narcolepsy with cataplexy	• Sleep attacks • Cataplexy Presence • 95% deficit of hypocretin in CSF or <110 pg/mL • HLA DQB1 * 0602 • MSLT: SL <8 min,> 2 SOREMPs
Narcolepsy without cataplexy	• attacks • Absence of cataplexy at the time of diagnosis • No deficiency of hypocretin • MSLT: SL <8 min,> 2 SOREMPs
Idiopathic hipersomnia	• Sleep attacks • Absence of cataplexy • MSLT: SL <8 min, <2 SOREMPs. • Hypersomnolence cannot be explained by other comorbid disorders or substance effects

Technique to Obtain MSLT Test

MSLT is a test performed in daily clinical practice at the laboratory of Sleep Disorders Unit at the General University Hospital of Castellón (Spain), accredited by the European Sleep Research Society (ESRS). Its main purpose is the study of hypersomnia.

The reaearch is carried out together with a PSG team from the Compumedics brand (Grael model). For the EEG record we use spoon electrodes (reusable) complemented with conductive paste to optimize the quality of the signals.

Another fundamental behaviour for the determination of REM phase is the presence of rapid eye movements; for its registration we use disposable skin electrodes, each located on the outer edge of each eye. With regard to the recording of muscle tone, three spoon electrodes placed on the mental and submental region are also used.

The assembly of the MSLT (recommendations Sleep 2005) [1] *should include:*

1. The EEG record: two paracentral electrodes (C3-C4) and two occipital electrodes (O1-O2) are placed after removing the rest of the electrodes used in the previous PSG, to improve patient comfort.
2. The two eye electrodes (EOG) are checked, each located 1 cm from the outer edge of the eye, one on the left side and the other on the right side.
3. Only 3 electrodes of the Mentonian electromyographic record (Chin) are maintained.
4. The electrodes (EMG) placed on the legs are removed.
5. Finally the room is prepared again in an environment that encourages sleep.

General Procedures Before the Implementation of an MSLT

The night prior to the completion of the MSLT, a PSG should be performed to basically assess sleep efficiency and rule out intrinsic sleep problems. For the PSG + MSLT, on the day of the study, it is recommended that patients wake up at the usual time and avoid consuming stimulants such as coffee or tea as well as sedatives such as alcohol and other substances that act at the level of the CNS and that may alter the test result.

Protocol for the Implementation of the MSLT

After PSG, patients should stay out of bed. Then they can wash, dress and have breakfast (avoiding stimulant drinks) It is also advised to avoid the use of screens. During this time patients will be monitored by the staff to confirm that they do not fall asleep or take any short naps. Around 1.5-2 hours after the end of the PSG, the first nap of the total of the 4-5 MSLT will begin, which must be carried out after a 2 hour interval between each of them.

PROTOCOL	PROCEDURE
PSG	At least 6-8 hours of sleep (> 70% efficiency)
Break 1,5-2 hours	
First Nap	**Do not fall asleep → 20 min record** **Sleep → 15 min (after 30 s any sleep phase).**
Break 1,5-2 hours	
Second Nap	Do not fall asleep → 20 min record Sleep → 15 min (after 30 s any sleep phase)
Break1,5-2 h	
Third Nap	Do not fall asleep → 20 min record Sleep → 15 min (after 30 s any sleep phase)
Break 1,5-2 h	
Fourth Nap	Do not fall asleep → 20 min record Sleep → 15 min (after 30 s any sleep phase)
Descanso 1,5-2 h	
Fifth Nap	Have you submitted 2 or more SOREMPS? YES: finish study NO: perform last nap

The test should guarantee patients the best conditions for sleep, that is, it should take place in a quiet ward, without noise or light and with a correct temperature.

Once this time interval has elapsed, patients must prepare again for the study that is the reason why they will be advised to wear comfortable clothes and then go back to bed, once the electrodes and the corresponding calibration have been connected.

In the hypothetical case that a patient does not fall asleep, the test ends 20 minutes after the light goes out.

In contrast, if a patient falls asleep or enters REM sleep, the test ends 15 minutes after the first 30-second sleep period.

As a general rule, four naps will be carried out, a fifth one completing the study if the entry into the REM is observed in one of the four preceding ones. In those patients who enter the REM stage two or more times during naps, the fifth nap could be omitted.

Interpretation of the Results of the MSLT

The criteria for the assessment of sleep onset are different from those corresponding to the interruption of the test.

- The sleep latency criteria applied in the MSLT are different from the typical definition of the start of the night sleep of PSG (phase N2 sleep or 10 min followed by sleep)
- Sleep latency in the MSLT: is the elapsed time (in minutes) from the time to turn off the lights until the first time of any sleep phase appears.

According to the evaluation criteria of Rechtschaffen and Kales, this implies that 16 seconds of sleep are enough to determine the beginning of sleep (that is, more than 50% of an epoch):

- The latency of REM sleep: it is valued as the minutes elapsed from the beginning of sleep until the appearance of the first time of REM sleep. The appearance of REM sleep at 10-15 minutes of sleep onset is called the REM period at the beginning of sleep (SOREMP, REM period of sleep onset).

- Other important parameter is the frequency of SOREMP. As previously mentioned, the presence of two or more SOREMP together with an average latency at the onset of short sleep is strongly related to the clinical suspicion of narcolepsy.
- The average sleep latency (in minutes) compared to the 4-5 MSLT is the measure of all the latencies of naps that are used characteristically to express the level of drowsiness. If it is less than 5 minutes it is considered pathological and around 5-10 minutes is more uncertain, although suggestive of hypersomnia.
- The result of MSLT is expressed in the form of a median sleep latency or in the form of an index of somnolence, which is the average latency subtracted from 100 and multiplied by 100% (correcting it when less than five naps are taken) [10]

Considerations Before the Realisation of MSLT

Since the level of sleepiness (the average sleep latency of the MSLT) is influenced by the quality and quantity of sleep in the previous night or weeks to the study, it is advisable to also register the sleep pattern with a sleep diary that should be filled the weeks before the study is performed. With special consideration in changes of the usual sleep habit (as in the case of shifts workers) and deterioration in the quality of sleep referred by the patient.

It is important to know the sedative or stimulant effects of the medications and their interruption for the correct interpretation of somnolence.

In some studies is descript the so-called effect of the last nap. This would occur in the 5th nap as a result of the anxiety generated before returning home to spend the day [11].

This effect could raise the average sleep latency during the day. The anticipation of going home can lengthen sleep latency or avoid the sleep in the last nap, it is recommended programming other activities that do not enhance awakening after the last test of latency.

The chronology of the circadian phase of MSLT influences the onset of REM sleep. This may appear in the latency tests performed early in the morning in people who normally sleep until late in the morning.

Patients with obstructive sleep apnea with more than 40 episodes per hour and very fragmented sleep can present short sleep average latencies during MSLT including some SOREMP (although the presence of 2 or more SOREMP is highly suggestive of narcolepsy) in these patients it is recommended to reevaluate them with a new study after correcting the underlying problem.

Although in patients with chronic insomnia, it could be thought, given that their nocturnal sleep is less, they should have short sleep latencies as a way of recovering lack of sleep. But it is true that it has been demonstrated that in these patients exist usually an excessive level of alertness. So the average sleep latencies are usually quite high (that is, greater than 15 minutes).

Drugs and Drowsiness

It is especially important to know about the treatments that usually takes the patient. As it is known, the depressant drugs increase somnolence and the stimulants of central nervous system reduce it. The hypnotics (especially from the group of benzodiazepines) accelerate the onset of sleep at bedtime and reduce the latency of return to sleep after an episode of awakening during the night. When administered at bedtime, those long-acting hypnotic continue to reduce sleep latency in the MSLT performed the day after administration. Antihistamine H1 drugs are associated with daytime drowsiness. Modafinil and methylphenidate increase the average of sleep latency [10].

DISCUSSION

The physiological sleepiness has a circadian rhythm. Also the daytime sleep attacks in the narcolepsy has a circadian rhythm, in serious cases, it must be recur every ninety minutes as a result of REM sleep pressure.

Precisely, the MSLT is based in this cyclic recurrence of daytime lapses into sleep and REM sleep pressure. If the excessive daytime sleepiness has a moderate grade, cause hyporeactivity and distractions. More serious forms induces an uncontrollable need to sleep, drop of sleep, amnesia and automatic behavior. The prevalence of the EDS is around 10-25% in general population [9] The polysomnography in addition to MSLT the next day, is the gold standard for the diagnosis of central disorders of hypersomnolence and for the differential diagnosis of others causes of hypersomnia (SAHS, RLS, etc) [6].

From a qualitative perspective, in NT1 and NT2 there must be excessive REM sleep pressure, expressed in the MSLT as entry quickly in this stage (SOREMPs).

From a quantitative point of view, narcolepsy is the sleep disorder that yields shorter scores in the MSL of the MSLT [12]; although the diagnostic criterion is less or equal than 8 minutes, it is usual in clinical practice to observe that the MSL is less than 5, even less than 3 minutes.

The SAHS can present even 2 SOREMPs in the MSLT, and the MSL for an apnea-hypopnea index (AHI) of 30/hour is between 6.03 and 7.52 minutes [13].

On the other hand, in idiopatic hypersomnia there is no REM sleep pressure, and the LPS usually has intermediate scores between Narcolepsy and SAHS [12]; MSLT in idiopatic hypersomnia is not sensitive or specific. It is logically essential to carry out the appropriate differential diagnosis with NT1 and NT2.

If it exists a strong clinical diagnostic suspicion and the MSLT is greater than 8 minutes, a MSLT ad libitum should be performed, leaving the patient to sleep freely (a total of 24 hours) after the PSG, and confirm a sleep period greater or equal than 660 minutes [14].

The different editions of the ICSD have included the MSLT as a fundamental clinical test for the diagnosis of narcolepsy, independently of the presence or absence of cataplexy.

However, recent studies have shown a marked instability in MSLT in NT2 over time [15, 16, 17], even indicating that many of the cases of positivity in the test could be attributed to circadian rhythm disorders or debit of sleep at the time of the test [17, 18] and in idiopatic hypersomnia [17, 19].

We present TLMS of longest published series in NT1:

- Pizza F et al. [20]. 79 patients. MSL: 3.23 ± 2.27 min. SOREMPs: 3.91 ± 1.28
- Um YH et al. [21]. 60 patients. MSL: 3.4 ± 0.4 min. SOREMPs: 3.6 ± 0.2
- Ruoff et al. [17]. 48 patients. MSL: 1.52 ± 0.93 min. SOREMPs: 3,56 ± 0.71
- Drakatos et al. [22]. 40 patients. MSL: 2.68 ± 1.90 min. There is no data of SOREMPs
- Kretzschmar et al. [12]. 35 patients. MSL: 1.9 ± 1.6 min. SOREMPs: 90% with 2 or more.
- Ramm et al. [23] 10 patients. MSL: 2.5 min (95% confidence interval 1.3-3.6)

We retrospectively analyzed the TLMS of patients with NT1 diagnosed in the Sleep

Unit of Universitary General Hospital of Castellón:

-40 pacientes. MSL: 3.468 ± 2.276 min. SOREMPs: median = 3

Our series is in line with the findings described in the literature, both of them, the MSL and the number of SOREMPS.

It is striking that in the longest series of patients with NT1 the SL is significantly greater than in the series with less number of patients.

CONCLUSION

1. The MSLT is fundamental for the diagnosis of NT1.
2. In NT1 the MSLT yields the lowest MSL and the highest number of SOREMPs within the hypersomnolence of central origin.
3. MSLT is repeatable in type 1 narcolepsy but not in type 2 narcolepsy.
4. The entity that shows findings similar to NT1 (very short SML and high number of SOREMPs) is the syndrome of insufficient sleep.
5. In cases of NT2, it is recommendable to repeat the MSLT to corroborate the findings.
6. In cases of suspected NT1 with doubtful cataplexy and without levels of hypocretin in CSF, MSLT should be repeated after recording sleep on the preceding days by actigraphy (not only by sleep schedule).

REFERENCES

[1] Littner MR., Kushida C., Wise M., Dávila DG., Morgenthaler T et al. (2005) Practice parameters for clinical use of the multiple sleep latency test and the maintenance of wakefulness test. *Sleep;* 28 (1): 113-21.

[2] Guillerminault C., Passouant P and Dement WC (Eds) (1975). *Narcolepsy*. (pp 1-689). News York: Spectrum.

[3] Richardson GS., Carskadon MA., Flagg W., Van den Hoed J., Dement WC et al. (1978) Excessive daytime sleepiness in man: Multiple sleep latency measurement in narcoleptic and control subjects. *Electroencephalography and Clinical Neurophysiology*; 45: 621-627.

[4] Mitler MM., Van den Hoed J., Carskadon MA., Richardson G., Park R, et al. (1979) REM sleep episodes during the Multiple Sleep

Latency Test in narcoleptic patients. *Electroencephalography and Clinical Neurophysiology*; 46: 479-481.

[5] Carskadon MA and Dement WC. (1975) Sleep studies on a 90-minute day. *ELectroencephalography and Clinical Neurophysiology*; 39: 145-155.

[6] American Academy of Sleep Medicine (2014*). The International Classification of Sleep Disorders (ICSD) diagnostic and coding manual.* 3rd ed. Westchester, IL: American Academy of Sleep Medicine.

[7] Andlauer O., Moore H., Jouhier L, et al. (2013) Nocturnal rapid eye movement sleep latency for identifying patients with narcolepsy/hypocretin deficiency. *JAMA Neurology*; 70 (7): 891-902.

[8] Cairns A., Bogan R. (2015) Prevalence and clinical correlates of a short onset REM period (SOREMP) during routine PSG. *Sleep;* 38 (10): 1575-1581.

[9] Reiter J., Katz E., Scammell TE., Maski K (2015) Usefulness of a nocturnal SOREMP for diagnosing narcolepsy with cataplexy in a pediatric population. *Sleep;* 38 (6): 859-865.

[10] Chokroverty S. (2016). Sleep Disorders Medicine. 3rd ed; New Jersey.

[11] Muza, R., Lykouras, D., & Rees, K. (2016). The utility of a 5(th) nap in multiple sleep latency test. *Journal of Thoracic Disease*, 8(2), 282–286. https://doi.org/10.3978/j.issn.2072-1439.2015.12.66.

[12] Kretzschmar U., Werth E., Sturzenegger C., Khatami R., Bassetti C et al. (2016) Which diagnostic findings in disorders with excessive daytime sleepiness are really helpful? A retrospective study. *Journal of Sleep Research*; 25: 307-31.

[13] Nam H., Lim J-S., Kim J-S., Lee K-J, Koo DL et al. (2016) Sleep perception in obstructive sleep apnea; a study using polysomnography and the multiple sleep latency test. *J Clin Neurol* 2016; 12 (2): 230-235.

[14] Billiard M, Sonka K. Idiopathic hypersomnia. (2016) *Sleep Med Rev*; 29: 23-33.

[15] Chenini, S., Evangelista, E., Jaussent, I., Doukkali, A., Dauvilliers, Y., Barateau, L., & Lopez, R. (2017). Test–Retest Reliability of the Multiple Sleep Latency Test in Central Disorders of Hypersomnolence. *Sleep*, 40(12). https://doi.org/10.1093/sleep/zsx164.

[16] Huang, Y. S., Guilleminault, C., Lin, C. H., Chen, C. H., Chin, W. C., & Chen, T. S. (2018). Multiple sleep latency test in narcolepsy type 1 and narcolepsy type 2: A 5-year follow-up study. *Journal of Sleep Research,* 27(5), 12700. https://doi.org/10.1111/jsr.12700.

[17] Ruoff C., Pizza F., Trotti LM., Sonka K., Vandi S et al. (2018) The MSLT is repeatable in narcolepsy type 1 but not narcolepsy type 2: a retrospective patient study. *J Clin Sleep Med*; 14 (1): 65-74.

[18] Goldbart A., Peppard P., Finn L., Ruoff C., Barnet J et al. (2014) Narcolepsy and predictors of positive MSLTs in the Wisconsin sleep cohort. *Sleep*; 37 (6): 1043-1051.

[19] Trotti LM., Staab BA, Rye DB. (2013) Test-retest reliability of the multiple sleep latency test in narcolepsy without cataplexy and idiopathic hypersomnia. *J Clin Sleep Med*; 9 (8): 789-795.

[20] Pizza F, Vandi S, Lloti M, Franceschini C, Liquori R et al. Nocturnal sleep dynamics identify narcolepsy type 1. *Sleep* 2015; 38 (8): 1277-84.

[21] Um YH, Kim TW, Jeong JH, Seo HJ, Han JH et al. A longitudinal follow-up study on multiple sleep latency test and body mass index of patients with narcolepsy type 1 in Korea. *J Clin Sleep Med* 2017; 13 (12): 1441-44.

[22] Drakatos P, Patel K, Thakrar C, Williams AJ, Kent BD et al. Sleep-stage sequencing of sleep-onset REM periods in MSLT predicts treatment response in patients with narcolepsy. *J Sleep Res* 2016; 25 (2): 203-210.

[23] Ramm M, Boentert M, Lojewsky N, Jafarpour A, Young P et al. Disease-specific attention impairment in disorders of chronic excessive daytime sleepiness. *Sleep Med* 2019; 53: 133-140.

In: New Research on Sleep …
Editor: Olivier Ratté
ISBN: 978-1-53616-882-2

Chapter 5

UPPER CERVICAL SPINE MORPHOLOGY: A NEW PHENOTYPIC SUBDIVISION OF PATIENTS WITH OBSTRUCTIVE SLEEP APNOEA

Liselotte Sonnesen*[*]*, PhD, Dr. Odont.
Department of Odontology, University of Copenhagen,
Copenhagen, Denmark

ABSTRACT

The main aim of this chapter is to describe the role of upper cervical spine morphology in diagnosis and treatment of patients with obstructive sleep apnea (OSA).

Pathological conditions of the cervical spine, such as osteoarthritis, cervical osteophytes and osteochondromas, have been reported in relation to OSA. Recently, the morphology of the upper cervical spine in patients with OSA has been described on two-dimensional lateral cephalograms and three-dimensional cone-beam computed tomography. The studies found that the prevalence and pattern of deviations of the upper cervical

[*] Corresponding Author's E-mail: alson@sund.ku.dk.

spine morphology in OSA was different compared to healthy controls. Furthermore, the facial profile including the cranial base was different in OSA patients with deviations of the upper cervical spine morphology compared to OSA patients without upper spine morphological deviations. In addition, the prevalence and pattern of upper cervical spine morphological deviations in OSA patients seem to affect the outcome of treatment with a mandibular advancement devise (MAD).

Accordingly, it is suggested that upper cervical spine morphology contributes to phenotypic differentiations between types of OSA and thereby to the diagnosis, subdivision and treatment of patients with OSA.

Keywords: cervical spine morphology, sleep apnoea, phenotype

INTRODUCTION

Obstructive sleep apnea (OSA) is by far the most common sleep-related breathing disorder, affecting 2-4% of the adult population, particularly males aged 60 years and older where the prevalence is 30-60% [1, 2]. OSA is defined as cessation of airflow with persistent respiratory effort, due to repeated anatomical obstruction or partial collapse of the oropharyngeal region, involving the soft palate, dorsum of the tongue and the posterior pharyngeal wall [1, 3]. The majority of the patients has symptoms such as loud snoring and excessive daytime sleepiness [4, 5]. Nightly choking or gasping, morning headache, memory loss, decreased concentration, increased irritability and nocturia are also reported [4, 6]. Thus OSA has consequences for the quality of life, working ability and traffic safety as well as co-morbidities as hypertension [4-7].

OSA is multifactorial with age, gender and body mass index (BMI) as predisposing factors [1, 3]. Authors agree that there are craniofacial morphological and postural characteristics in OSA patients such as reduced posterior airway space, abnormally long soft palate, low position of the hyoid bone and an extended head posture [8, 9].

The upper airway is normally maintained by the bony and cartilaginous structures surrounding the naso- and oropharynx. Located posterior to the pharynx, the cervical spine is composed of seven vertebrae that provide full range of motion to the neck through articulations with the occiput and between the vertebrae. Some studies have been performed on the relationship between the cervical spine and OSA. Pathological conditions as osteoarthritis of the cervical spine [10-13], cervical osteophytes [14-16] and osteochondromas [17, 18] have been reported in relation to OSA patients. Recently, the morphology of the upper cervical spine in patients with OSA has been described on two-dimensional lateral cephalograms [19, 20] and three-dimensional cone-beam computed tomography (CBCT) [21, 22].

Due to the cervical spine's close association with the upper airway this chapter will focus on the role of the morphology of the upper cervical spine in the diagnosis and treatment in patients with OSA.

UPPER SPINE MORPHOLOGY

Morphological deviations of the upper cervical spine have previously been described in relation to craniofacial syndromes and cleft lip and palate. Craniosynostosis syndromes, for example, Pfeiffer's, Crouzon's and Apert's syndromes, showed deviations such as fusion anomalies [23-27]. Furthermore, deviations of the upper cervical spine morphology were seen in Saethre-Chotzen, Klippel-Feil, Turner, Down syndromes and patients with hypophosphatemic rickets [28-34]. Also, upper spine morphological deviations have been closely investigated in patients with cleft lip and/or palate [35-40]. Recently, upper spine morphological deviations are also found to be associated with severe malocclusion traits and the craniofacial profile [41-48].

Specific pathological conditions of the upper spine such as osteoarthritis [10-13], cervical osteophytes [14-16] and osteochondromas [17, 18] have been reported in relation to OSA patients. These conditions associated with OSA may be due to a direct relationship to the pharyngeal dimensions resulting in a decrease in the pharyngeal airway dimensions [10-18]. These pathological conditions are often parts of genereal syndromes that cause OSA [49] and thereby make it diffecult to distinguish if it is the general syndrome or the cervical spine pathology that result in a descreased airway dimension. However, only few studies have investigated the morphology of the upper cervical spine in patients with obstructive sleep apnoea [19-22], which wil be described in the following.

Upper Spine Morphology in Patients with Obstructive Sleep Apnoea

Definition of Upper Cervical Spine Morphology

The upper cervical spine morphology can be obtained from conventional 2-dimentional (2D) lateral cephalograms or from 3-dimentional (3D) cone beam computed tomography (CBCT). One method to describe the upper cervical spine morphology on either lateral cephalograms or on CBCT is by visual assessment of the first five cervical vertebral units as referred to in this chapter. The morphological deviations are divided into two categories "Posterior arch deficiency" and "Fusion anomalies" [36, 41, 50]:

1) Posterior arch deficiency consisted of *partial cleft*: failure of the posterior part of the neural arch to fuse and *dehiscence*: failure of part of a vertebral unit to develop.
2) Fusion anomalies consisted of *fusion*: fusion of one unit with another at the vertebral bodies, articulation facets, neural arch or transverse processes, *block fusion*: fusion of more than 2 units at the vertebral bodies, articulation facets, neural arch or transverse processes and *occipitalization*: assimilation, either partially or completely of the atlas (C1) with the occipital bone.

The method has previously been validated and the inter- and intra-observer agreement on the lateral cephalogram and on CBCT was found to be very good [21, 42]. Furthermore, when the occurrence of morphological deviations of the upper cervical spine on lateral cephalograms and on CBCTs was compared no statistically significant differences were found and the agreement between the occurrence of upper cervical spine morphological deviations seen on lateral cephalograms and CBCTs was good [21].

Thus, lateral cephalograms (already available after indication in connection with e.g., treatment planning) are considered sufficient for identifying morphological deviations in the upper cervical spine. But for a more accurate diagnosis and location of the deviations a CBCT is required [21].

Prevalence and Pattern of Upper Spine Morphology

Previous studies have shown that morphological deviations in the upper cervical spine in terms of fusion anomalies and posterior arch deficiency evaluated on 2D lateral cephalograms and 3D CBCT occurred significantly more often in OSA patients compared to healthy controls [19, 21].

Fusion anomalies in OSA patients occurred in 32-46% as *fusions*: either between the second and third vertebrae, between the third and fourth vertebrae, or between the fourth and fifth cervical vertebrae; *block fusions*: fusions either between the second, third, or fourth vertebrae, between the second, third, fourth, and fifth vertebrae, or between the third, fourth, and fifth vertebrae; *occipitalization* in combination with fusions, block fusions or as a single deviation [19, 21] (Figure 1).

Posterior arch deficiency in OSA patients occurred in 5-14% as *partial cleft* of the first cervical vertebra or *dehiscence* of the third cervical vertebra and the fourth cervical vertebra [19, 21] (Figure 1).

The pattern of morphological deviations in the upper spine seen in OSA patients are more severe and occurred more caudally than seen in healthy subjects (Figure 1) and in orthodontic patients with severe malocclusion [41-48].

Occipitalization, block fusion and dehiscence were the phenotypes, which were characteristic of sleep apnea (Figure 1).

It is presumed that the pattern and location of upper cervical spine morphological deviations is connected to different locations of neural crest cell migration along the body axis [51].

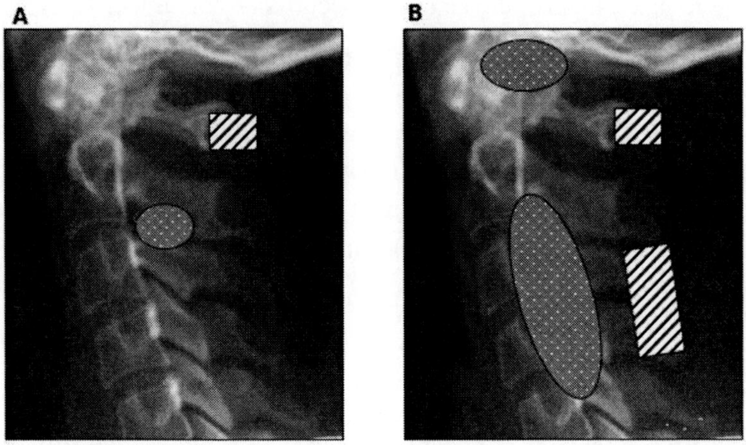

Figure 1. Radiological illustration of a normal upper cervical spine with indications of the pattern and location of observed morphological deviations of the upper cervical spine in **A**: Healthy adult subjects and **B**: Patients with obstructive sleep apnoea. Grey with dots indicate the pattern and location of fusion anomalies. White with stripes indicate the pattern and location of posterior arch deficiency.

Accordingly, it is hypothesized that the level of pharyngeal obstruction in sleep apnea is associated with the caudally/cranially positioned cervical spine malformation.

Caracterictics of OSA Patients with Upper Spine Morphological Deviations

Not only was a specific pattern of morphological deviations in the upper cervical spine in patients with OSA found, but head posure and the craniofacial morphology seem also to be different in OSA patients with upper spine morphological deviations.

OSA patients with morphological deviations in the upper spine had a significantly more backward and curved neck posture compared to OSA patients without upper spine deviations [22]. The findings were in agreement with previous studies where an association was found between morphological deviations in the upper spine and posture of the head and neck in healthy adults [46] and in children with class II malocclusion [47].

Furthermore, the craniofacial profile of OSA patients with upper spine morphological deviations was significantly different from the craniofacial profile in OSA patients without deviations in the upper spine [20]. A long and retrognathic facial profile together with an extended head posture was characteristic of OSA patients with upper spine morphological deviations.

In addition, OSA patients with morphological deviations in the upper spine may respond poorer to mandibular advancement devise (MAD) treatment compared to OSA patients without morphological deviations in the upper spine [52].

The findings indicate that the aetiology in OSA patients with morphological deviations in the upper spine is characterised by other factors or combinations of different factors than in OSA patients without upper spine morphological deviations [19, 21, 22, 52]. The morphological deviations in the upper cervical spine may therefore contribute to phenotypic differentiations between types of OSA and thereby to the diagnosis, subdivision and treatment of patients with OSA [19, 21, 22, 52].

The association between OSA and morphological deviations in the upper cervical spine found in previous studies [19-22, 52] may be explained by the relationship between the upper spine morphology and pharyngeal airway dimensions. But no significant differences in the pharyngeal airway dimensions between patients with and without upper spine morphological deviations have been found [22] indicating that no direct relationship between the upper spine morphology and pharyngeal airway dimensions exists. However, the association between OSA and upper spine morphological deviations may be due to the direct relationship between upper spine morphological deviations and head posture [22] as an extended head posture were associated with increased upper airway dimensions in OSA patients [9, 22, 53-58].

Another explanation for the association between OSA and morphological deviations in the upper spine especially the interrelationship between the upper spine and the craniofacial morphology may be found in the early embryological development of these structures [59]. It has been documented that the development of the body axis is regulated by the notochord [60]. It is also well known that the notochord runs in its full extent from the sacral region to the sella turcica in the posterior part of the cranial base to which the jaws are attached [51]. A deviation in the development of the notochord may influence the surrounding bone tissue in the spine as well as in the posterior part of the cranial base and thereby the development of the jaws. The shared origin of the spine and posterior part of the cranial base is the basis for the hypothesis of associations between the spine and the cranial base to which the jaws are attached [61, 62].

So far, the complex aetiology of OSA is not fully understood and the explanation for the association between upper spine morphological deviations and OSA is still unknown.

However, the findings indicated that the aetiology in OSA patients with morphological deviations in the upper spine is characterized by other factors or combinations of different factors than in OSA patients without upper spine morphological deviations and that upper spine morphological deviations therefore may influence the MAD treatment outcome in OSA patient [19, 21, 22, 52]. Therefore, it may be suggested that OSA patients with upper spine morphological deviations should be treated with CPAP and OSA patients without upper spine morphological deviations should be treated with MAD. This recommendation should be investigated further [22].

Conclusion

Morphological deviations in the upper cervical spine occurred significantly more often in patients with OSA compared to healthy controls and occipitalization, block fusion and dehiscence were the phenotypes, which were characteristic of OSA. OSA patients with upper spine morphological deviations were characterized by an extended head and neck posture and a long-face craniofacial morphology. Furthermore, OSA patients with upper spine morphological deviations may respond poorer to mandibular advancement devise treatment. Accordingly, upper cervical spine morphology contributes to phenotypic differentiations between types of OSA and thereby to the diagnosis, subdivision and treatment of patients with OSA.

References

[1] Prisant, L. M., Dillard, T. A., Blanchard, A. R. Obstructive sleep apnea syndrome. *J. Clin. Hypertens.,* (Greenwich) 2006; 8:746 - 750.

[2] Wolkove, N., Elkholy, O., Baltzan, M., Palayew, M. (2007) Sleep and aging: 1.Sleep disorders commonly found in older people. *CMAJ,* 2007; 176:1299 - 1304.

[3] Guilleminault, C., Tilkian, A., Dement, W. C. The sleep apnea syndromes. *Annu. Rev. Med.,* 1976; 27:465 - 484.

[4] Balachandran, J. S., Patel, S. R. In the clinic. Obstructive sleep apnea. *Ann. Intern. Med.,* 2014; 161:ITC1.

[5] Ngiam, J., Balasubramaniam, R., Darendeliler, M. A., Cheng, A. T., Waters, K., Sullivan, C. E. Clinical guidelines for oral appliance therapy in the treatment of snoring and obstructive sleep apnea. *Aust. Dent. J.,* 2013; 58:408 - 419.

[6] Epstein, L. J., Kristo, D., Strollo, Jr., P. J., Friedman, N. Clinical guideline for the evaluation, management and long-term care of obstructive sleep apnea in adults. *J. Clin. Sleep Med.,* 2009; 5:263 - 276.

[7] Jordan, A. S., McSharry, D. G., Malhotra, A. Adult obstructive sleep apnoea. *Lancet,* 2014; 383:736 - 747.

[8] Neelapu, B. C., Kharbanda, O. P., Sardana, H. K., Balachandran, R., Sardana, V., Kapoor, P., Gupta, A., Vasamsetti, S. Craniofacial and upper airway morphology in adult obstructive sleep apnea patients: A systematic review and meta-analysis of cephalometric studies. *Sleep Med. Rev.*, 2016. DOI: 10.1016/j.smrv.2016.01.007.

[9] Solow, B., Skov, S., Ovesen, J., Norup, P. W., Wildschiødtz, G. Airway dimensions and head posture in obstructive sleep apnoea. *Eur. J. Orthod.,* 1996; 18(6):571 - 579.

[10] Shoda, N., Seichi, A., Takeshita, K., Chikuda, H., Ono, T., Oka, H., Kawaguchi, H., Nakamura, K. Sleep apnea in rheumatoid arthritis patients with occipitocervical lesions: the prevalence and associated radiographic features. *Eur. Spine J.,* 2009 Jun.; 18(6):905 - 10. [doi: 10.1007/s00586-009-0975].

[11] Nguyen, H. V., Ludwig, S. C., Silber, J., Gelb, D. E., Anderson, P. A., Frank, L., Vaccaro, A. R. Rheumatoid arthritis of the cervical spine. *The Spine Journal,* 2004 May; 4(3): 329 - 34. [doi.org/ 10.1016/j.spinee.2003.10.006].

[12] Drossaers-Bakker, K. W., Hamburger, H. L., Bongartz, E. B., Dijkmans, B. A., Van Soesbergen, R. M. (1998) Sleep apnoea caused by rheumatoid arthritis. *Br. J. Rheumatol.,* 1998 Aug.; 37(8): 889 - 94.

[13] Sonnesen, L., Petersson, A., Wiese, M., Jensen, K. E., Svanholt, P., Bakke, M. 2017. Osseous osteoarthritic like changes and joint mobility of the temporomandibular joints and upper cervical spine is there a relation? *Oral Surg. Oral Med. Oral Pathol. Oral Radiol.,* 123(2):273 - 279.

[14] Eyigor, H., Selcuk, O. T., Osma, U., Koca, R., Yilmaz, M. D. Cervical osteophytes: a rare cause of obstructive sleep apnea. *J. Craniofac. Surg.,* 2012 Sep.; 23(5):e444 - 6. [doi: 10.1097/ SCS.0b013e318260e9ea].

[15] Ando, E., Ogawa, T., Shigeta, Y., Hirai, S., Ikawa, T., Ishikawa, C., Nejima, J. A case of obstructive sleep apnoea with anterior cervical osteophytes. *J. Oral Rehabil.,* 2009 Oct.; 36(10):776 - 80. [doi: 10.1111/j.1365-2842.2009.01984].

[16] Fuerderer, S., Eysel-Gosepath, K., Schroder, U., Delank, K. S., Eysel, P. Retro-pharyngeal obstruction in association with osteophytes of the cervical spine. *J. Bone Joint Surg. Br.,* 2004 Aug.; 86(6): 837 - 40.

[17] Wang, V., Chou, D. Anterior C1–2 osteochondroma presenting with dysphagia and sleep apnea. *J. Clin. Neurosci.,* 2009 Apr.; 16(4):581 - 2. [doi: 10.1016/j.jocn.2008.05.024].

[18] Yoshida, T., Matsuda, H., Horiuchi, C., Taguchi, T., Nagao, J., Aota, Y., Honda, A., Tsukuda, M. A case of osteochondroma of the atlas causing obstructive sleep apnea syndrome. *Acta Otolaryngol.,* 2006 Apr.; 126(4): 445 - 8. [doi:10.1080/00016480500416793].

[19] Sonnesen, L., Petri, N., Kjaer, I., Svanholt, P. Cervical column morphology in adult patients with obstructive sleep apnoea. *Eur. J. Orthod.,* 2008; 30: 521 - 6.

[20] Svanholt, P., Petri, N., Wildschiødtz, G., Sonnesen, L., Kjaer, I. Associations between craniofacial morphology, head posture, and cervical vertebral body fusions in men with sleep apnoea. *Am. J. Orthod. Dentofac. Orthop.,* 2009 Jun.; 135(6):702.e1 - 9; discussion 702 - 3. [doi: 10.1016/j.ajodo.2009.02.011].

[21] Sonnesen, L., Jensen, K. E., Petersson, A. R., Petri, N., Berg, S., Svanholt, P. Cervical vertebral column morphology in patients with obstructive sleep apnoea assessed using lateral cephalograms and cone beam CT. A comparative study. *Dentomaxillofac. Radiol.,* 2013; 42(6):20130060. [doi: 10.1259/dmfr.20130060].

[22] Sonnesen, L., Petersson, A., Berg, S., Svanholt, P. 2017. Pharyngeal Airway Dimensions and Head Posture in Obstructive Sleep Apnea Patients with and without Morphological Deviations in the Upper Cervical Spine. *J. Oral Maxillofac. Res.,* 30;8(3):e4.

[23] Hemmer, K. M., McAlister, W. H., Marsh, J. L. Cervical spine anomalies in the craniosynostosis syndromes. *Cleft Palate J.,* 1987; 24(4):328 - 333.

[24] Kreiborg, S., Barr, Jr. M., Cohen, Jr. M. M. Cervical spine in the Apert syndrome. *Am. J. Med. Genet.,* 1992; 43(4):704 - 708.

[25] Anderson, P. J., Hall, C. M., Evans, R. D., Jones, B. M., Harkness, W., Hayvard, R. D. The cervical spine in Pfeiffer's syndrome. *J. Craniofac. Surg.,* 1996; 7(4):275 - 279.

[26] Anderson, P. J., Hall, C., Evans, R. D., Jones, B. M., Harkness, W. J., Hayward, R. D. The cervical spine in Crouzon syndrome. *Spine,* 1997; 22(4): 402 - 405.

[27] Thompson, D. N. P., Slaney, S. F., Hall, C. M., Shaw, D., Jones, B. M., Hayward, R. D. Congenital cervical spinal fusion: a study in Apert syndrome. *Pediatr. Neurosurg.,* 1996; 25(1):22 - 27.

[28] Anderson, P. J., Hall, C. M., Evans, R. D., Hayward, R. D., Harkness, W. J., Jones, B. M. The cervical spine in Saethre-Chotzen syndrome. *Cleft Palate Craniofac. J.,* 1997; 34(1):79 - 82.

[29] Frost, M., Huffer, W. E., Sze, C. I., Badesch, D., Cajade-Law, A. G., Kleinschmidt-Demasters, B. K. Cervical spineabnormalities in Down syndrome. *Clin. Neuropathol.,* 1999; 18(5);250 - 259.

[30] Trusen, A., Beissert, M., Collmann, H., Darge, K. The pattern of skeletal anomalies in the cervical spine, hands and feet in patients with Saethre-Chotzen syndrome and Muenketype mutation. *Pediatric Radiology,* 2003; 33(3):168 - 172.

[31] Samartzis, D., Herman, J., Lubicky, J. P., Shen, F. H. Classification of congenitally fused cervical patterns in Klippel-Feil patients: epidemiology and role in the development ofcervical spine-related symptoms. *Spine,* 2006; 31(21):E798 - E804. DOI:10.1097/01.brs.0000239222.36505.46.

[32] Shen, F. H., Samartzis, D., Herman, Lubicky J. P. Radiographic assessment of segmental motion at the atlantoaxial junction in the Klippel-Feil patient. *Spine,* 2006; 31(2):171 - 177.

[33] Gjørup, H., Sonnesen, L., Beck-Nielsen, S. S., Haubek, D. Upper spine morphology in hypophosphatemic rickets and healthy controls: a radiographic study. *Eur. J. Orthod.,* 2014; 36(2):217 - 225.

[34] Michelsen, T., Brusgaard, P., Sonnesen, L. Klippel-Feil: A syndrome in the occipital-cervical spine field and its dentofacial manifestations. *World J. Stomatol.,* 2015; 20(2):81 - 86.

[35] Ross, R. B., Lindsay, W. K. The cervical vertebrae as a factor in etiology of cleft palate. *Cleft Palate J.,* 1965; 36:273 - 281.

[36] Sandham, A. Cervical vertebral anomalies in cleft lip and palate. *Cleft Palate J.,* 1986; 23(3):206 - 214.

[37] Horswell, B. B. The incidence and relationship of cervical spine anomalies in patients with cleft lip and/or palate. *J. Oral Maxillofac. Surg.,* 1991; 49(7):693 - 697.

[38] Hoenig, J. F., Schoener, W. F. Radiological survey of the cervical spine in cleft lip and palate. *Dentomaxillofac. Radiol.,* 1992; 21(1): 36 - 39.

[39] Ugar, D. A., Semb, G. The prevalence of anomalies of the upper cervical vertebrae in subjects with cleft lip, cleft palate,or both. *Cleft Palate Craniofac. J.,* 2001; 38(5):498 - 503.

[40] Rajion, Z. A., Townsend, G. C., Netherway, D. J. et al. A three dimensional computed tomographic analysis of the cervical spine in unoperated infants with cleft lip and palate. *Cleft Palate Craniofac. J.,* 2006; 43(5):513 - 518.

[41] Sonnesen, L. Associations between the Cervical Vertebral Column and Craniofacial Morphology. *Int. J. Dent.,* 2010; 2010:295728. DOI: 0.1155/2010/295728.

[42] Sonnesen, L., Kjaer, I. Cervical column morphology in patients with skeletal Class III malocclusion and mandibular overjet. *Am. J. Orthod. Dentofacial. Orthop.,* 2007; 132(4): 427.e7 - 12. DOI:10.1016/j.ajodo.2007.01.019.

[43] Sonnesen, L., Kjaer, I. Cervical vertebral body fusions in patients with skeletal deep bite. *Eur. J. Orthod.,* 2007; 29(5):464 - 470.

[44] Sonnesen, L., Kjaer, I. Anomalies of the cervical vertebrae in patients with skeletal Class II malocclusion and horizontal maxillary overjet. *Am. J. Orthod. Dentofacial. Orthop.,* 2008; 133(2):188.e15 - 20. DOI: 10.1016/j.ajodo.2007.07.018.

[45] Sonnesen, L., Kjaer, I. Cervical column morphology in patients with skeletal open bite. *Orthodontics and Craniofacial Research,* 2008; 11(1):17 - 23.

[46] Sonnesen, L., Pedersen, C. E., Kjær, I. Cervical column morphology related to head posture, cranial base angle, and condylar malformation. *Eur. J. Orthod.,* 2007; 29(4):398 - 403.

[47] Arntsen, T., Sonnesen, L. Cervical vertebral column morphology related to craniofacial morphology and head posture in preorthodontic children with Class II malocclusion and horizontal maxillary overjet. *Am. J. Orthod. Dentofacial. Orthop.,* 2011; 140(1):e1 - 7.

[48] Kim, P., Sarauw, M. T., Sonnesen, L. Cervical vertebral column morphology and head posture in preorthodontic patients with anterior open bite. *Am. J. Orthod. Dentofacial. Orthop.,* 2014; 145(3):359 - 366.

[49] Khan, A., Than, K. D., Chen, K. S., Wang, A. C., La Marca, F., Park, P. Sleep apnea and cervical spine pathology. *Eur. Spine J.,* 2014 Mar.; 23(3):641 - 7. [doi: 10.1007/s00586-013-3046-4].

[50] Sonnesen, L. Head posture and upper spine morphology in relation to the craniofacial profile and orofacial function. In: Curran, S. A., editor. *Posture: Types, Exercises and Health Effects.* Nova Science Publishers, Inc. USA.;2014.Chapter 3, p. 43 - 55.

[51] Kjaer, I. Neuroosteology. *Crit. Rev. Oral Biol. Med.,* 1999; 9:224 - 244.

[52] Svanholt, P., Petri, N., Wildschiødtz, G., Sonnesen, L. Influence of craniofacial and upper spine morphology on mandibular advancement device treatment outcome in patients with obstructive sleep apnoea: a pilot study. *Eur. J. Orthod.,* 2015; 37:391 - 397.

[53] Tong, M., Sakakibara, H., Xia, X., Suetsugu, S. Compensatory head posture changes in patients with obstructive sleep apnea. *J. Tongji Med. Univ.,* 2000; 20(1):66 - 69.

[54] Choi, J. K., Goldman, M., Koyal, S., Clark, G. Effect of Jaw and Head Position on Airway Resistance in Obstructive Sleep Apnea. *Sleep Breath,* 2000; 4(4):163 - 168.

[55] Tangugsorn, V., Krogstad, O., Espeland, L., Lyberg, T. Obstructive sleep apnea (OSA): a cephalometric analysis of severe and non-severe OSA patients. Part I: Multiple comparison of cephalometric variables. *Int. J. Adult Orthodon. Orthognath. Surg.,* 2000; 15(2):139 - 152.

[56] Ozbek, M. M., Miyamoto, K., Lowe, A. A., Fleetham, J. A. .Natural head posture, upper airway morphology and obstructive sleep apnoea severity in adults. *Eur. J. Orthod.,* 1998; 20(2):133 - 143.

[57] Solow, B., Ovesen, J., Nielsen, P. W., Wildschiødtz, G., Tallgren, A. Head posture in obstructive sleep apnoea. *Eur. J. Orthod.,* 1993; 15(2): 107 - 114.

[58] Tangugsorn, V., Skatvedt, O., Krogstad, O., Lyberg, T. Obstructive sleep apnoea: a cephalometric study. Part I. Cervico-craniofacial skeletal morphology. *Eur. J. Orthod.,* 1995; 17(1):45 - 56.

[59] Kjaer, I. Human prenatal craniofacial development related to brain development under normal and pathological conditions. *Acta Odontol. Scand.*, 1995; 53:135 - 143.

[60] Kjaer, I., Kjær, T. W., Græm, N. Ossification sequence of occipital bone and vertebrae in human fetuses. *J. Craniofac. Genet. Dev. Biol.,* 1993; 13:83 - 88.

[61] Sonnesen, L., Nolting, D., Kjaer, K. W., Kjaer, I. Association between the development of the body axis and the craniofacial skeleton studied by immunohistochemical analyses using collagen II, Pax9, Pax1, and Noggin antibodies. *Spine,* (Phila Pa 1976). 2008; 33(15):1622 - 6.

[62] Sonnesen, L., Nolting, D., Engel, U., Kjaer, I. Cervical vertebrae, cranial base, and mandibular retrognathia in human triploid fetuses. *Am. J. Med. Genet. A,* 2009; 149A(2):177 - 187.

In: New Research on Sleep
Editor: Olivier Ratt
ISBN: 978-1-53616-882-2

Chapter 6

SNORING SOUNDS AND OROPHARYNGEAL SOFT TISSUES: SOME TYPICAL PROPERTIES FOR DETECTION AND DIAGNOSIS OF OBSTRUCTIVE SLEEP APNEA

***Tsuyoshi Mikami*[1,*], *Hirotaka Takahashi*[2,†] *and Kazuya Yonezawa*[3,‡]**
[1]Department of Computer Science and Engineering,
National Institute of Technology, Tomakomai College,
Tomakomai, Hokkaido, Japan
[2]Department of Information and Management Systems Engineering,
Nagaoka University of Technology, Nagaoka, Niigata, Japan
[3]Department of Clinical Research,
Hakodate National Hospital, Hakodate, Hokkaido, Japan

Abstract

As it has been reported that some serious traffic accidents are caused by sleep apnea syndrome (SAS), detection and diagnosis of SAS have increasingly become important in recent years. In this chapter, the authors present some useful knowledge obtained by analyzing the acoustic

[*]Corresponding Author's E-mail: mikami@tomakomai-ct.ac.jp.
[†]Corresponding Author's E-mail: hirotaka@kjs.nagaokaut.ac.jp.
[‡]Corresponding Author's E-mail: kyonezaw@hnh.hosp.go.jp.

properties of snoring sounds and the morphological properties of oropharyngeal soft tissues. Snoring sounds and oropharyngeal soft tissues are directly or indirectly related to the severity of SAS. The sections are organized as follows. The first section provides fundamental knowledge regarding snoring sounds and oropharyngeal soft tissues for detection and diagnosis of Obstructive SAS (OSAS) and introduces related studies. The second section describes the differences among acoustic properties of snoring sounds produced by different respiratory routes; oral, nasal, and oronasal inhalation. Since nasal congestion and open mouth during sleep are often regarded as risk factors of OSAS, recognizing such differences is a key to identifying which part is easy to be corrupted when apnea occurs. The third section demonstrates that morphological properties of tongue and soft palate are related to the severity of OSAS. By using the results of our quantitative analysis of MRIs, you can recognize the typical shapes of these soft tissues found in severe OSAS patients. The fourth section focuses on some kinds of unique snores; post-apneic snores. In general, these snores are said to be gasp-like sounds intrinsic to OSAS. But they have not been analyzed in detail, because their nonlinear and nonstationary properties make it difficult to properly calculate the spectra using traditional signal processing techniques. In this section, Hilbert-Huang transform (HHT) designed for analyzing this type of signals is applied to post-apneic snores and their nonlinearity and nonstationarity are quantitatively clarified based on the HHT spectra. Finally, the last section is devoted to a conclusion and future works.

Keywords: snoring sound, tongue morphology, MRI, signal processin Hilbert-Huang transform

INTRODUCTION

Detection and Diagnosis of Obstructive Sleep Apnea

An Obstructive Sleep Apnea (OSAS) is a sleep disorder that includes cessatic or significant decrease in airflow due to the corruption of the oropharyngeal so tissues during sleep. As it has been reported that some serious traffic acciden are caused by sleep apnea syndrome (SAS), detection and diagnosis of SA have increasingly become important in recent years.

Nowadays, a polysomnography (PSG) is a gold standard method for dete tion and diagnosis of SAS and is widely used in common. It consists of tens contact sensors such as EEG, ECG, EMG, EOG, thermistor, pulse oximetry, and so on. These sensors should be equipped on the patients body so as to estimate Apnea/Hypopnea Index (AHI), which is used for an objective index indicating the severity of SAS. But PSG requires patients to sleep in a hospital all night, so in some cases they cannot sleep as deeply as usual and the severity is often underestimated due to the first night effect [1]. In order to avoid this effect, it is better to record the biosignals in the same room at the hospital for several consecutive nights, but actually the several times of recording are done only when some irregular results are obviously identified. Normally, the PSG data through the first night are used for medical diagnosis.

Other methods for detection and diagnosis of SAS are nasal ventilation test, Mallampati test (visual recognition of pharyngeal structure), X-ray cephalometry, upper airway MRI and simple monitoring devices equipped with one or two sensors. Since these are mainly used for the initial screening before PSG, it is important to modify them or to develop a new method for precise screening and diagnosis of SAS. For this purpose, this chapter focuses on the acoustic properties of snoring sounds and the morphological properties of oropharyngeal soft tissues.

Why Snores and Soft Tissues?

Snoring is one of the typical symptoms of OSAS, but they are not so much used for the diagnosis. But some of the characteristics of snoring sounds in OSAS patients have been empirically reported so far. Snoring sounds of OSAS patients are known to be very loud and accompanied by gasps or choking. The acoustic properties have not been completely clarified quantitatively on account of its complicated mechanism. Since it is, however, easy to record snoring sounds with only a microphone and a sound recorder, many researchers have explore the possibility for the use of medical diagnosis.

Snoring is a vibration of oropharyngeal soft tissues provoked by inhalation. The enlargement of the tissues directly affects the sound properties and makes the airway narrower. But in some cases a certain type of morphological properties, not the enlargement, may lead to the airway obstruction. In order to identify such properties, X-ray or MR images has naturally been adopted so far.

Soft tissues are clearly recognized in MR images in comparison with X-ray images. In addition, three-dimensional anatomical features can be evaluated.

Thus, many researchers have focused on some 3-dimensional features of th oropharyngeal organization to clarify the relation to the severity of OSAS, b those conventional studies have only analyzed quite simple features. The mo detailed morphological analysis is expected by the use of some image proces ing techniques.

Evaluation of Snoring Sounds in Conventional Studies

Many medical researchers have analyzed snoring sounds so far in an attem to clarify the difference between the acoustic properties of snoring sounds i patients with and without Obstructive Sleep Apnea Syndrome (OSAS) [2] [[4] [5] [6] [7] [8].

Perez-Padilla et al. [2] firstly demonstrated that apnea patients had residu energy at 1 kHz whereas the nonapneic snorers did not. So, they said that th ratio of power above 800Hz to power below 800Hz could be used to separa snorers from OSAS patients. Fiz et al. [3] found the presence of a fundament frequency and several harmonics in snoring sounds of many simple snorers an a low frequency peak with the second energy scattered on a narrower band an without clearly identified harmonics in those of OSAS patients.

On the other hand, Herzog et al. [4] showed that patients with primar snoring revealed peak intensities between 100 and 300 Hz, whereas OSAS p tients showed peak intensities above 1 kHz. The PSG and BMI correlated wi peak intensity of the power spectrum. Hara et al. [5] have reported that th sound spectrum of the simple snorers shows a single peak at a lower frequenc whereas the snores of OSAS patients show multiple power peaks of vario amplitudes.

Some researchers have focused on the formant analysis generally adopted i speech recognition technique. Sola-Soler et al. [6] have showed significant di ferences in formant frequencies variability between simple snorers and OSA patients even when non-postapneic snores were considered. Ng et al. [7] hav also found quantitative differences in formant frequencies between apneic an benign snorers by the use of a Linear Predictive Coding (LPC) technique. A neic snorers exhibit higher formant frequencies than benign snorers, especial F1, which can be related to the pathology of OSAS. Emoto et al. [8] focuse on the standard deviation of the estimated formant frequencies (F1) in snorir episodes over 6 hours, which is relatively higher in OSAS patients than in sin ple (benign) snorers.

These studies have analyzed snoring sounds of simple snorers and those of apnea patients using FFT or LPC techniques, but their results are quite various. Thus, many researchers have still tried to clarify quantitative differences between acoustic properties of benign snores and those of apneic ones.

Evaluation of Soft Tissues in Conventional Studies

According to the MR images, it can be found that the upper airway in OSAS patients is narrower than those in benign persons. Especially, the enlargement of the upper airway soft tissues such as soft palate, uvula, tongue, and tonsils are the main factors of airway obstruction. Morphological features of them have been quantitatively analyzed so far by the use of cephalogram [9] [10] [11] [12], and MR images [13] [14] [15] [16] [17] [18].

Cephalogram is the measurement of the human head by X-ray imaging and is used to gauge the size and spacial relationships of the teeth, jaws, and cranium. Recently, it has been reported that the distance from the mandibular plane to the hyoid bone (MP-H) and the length of the soft palate (PNS-P) are highly correlated with AHI. In X-ray images, hard tissues such as bones or cartilage can clearly be recognized. However, since the soft tissues are not so clearly recognized in X-ray images, much experience in image diagnosis is necessary to visually determine the gaging points.

In the case of MR images, soft tissues are clearly recognized and three-dimensional evaluation is also practicable. In conventional studies, the volume of the tongue and the airway capacity [14] [18], fat volume [16], and the length around the neck [16] [17] have been analyzed quantitatively. Arens et al. [15] evaluated the relation of the length from the mandible bone to the clivus with AHI in a little more detail than conventional studies, but the detailed morphological features of the soft tissues have not sufficiently been analyzed so far.

Table 1 shows some morphological features of the soft tissue in the upper airway (but BMI is not) and the correlation coefficients with AHI, which have been reported in conventional studies [9] [10] [11] [12].

Table 1. Correlation between AHI and morphologic properties in conventional studies

Feature	Method	Corr. Coef.	p-value	Literature
PNS-P	Cephalogram	0.194	0.011	Kitamura et al. [9]
		0.240		Yu et al. [10]
MP-H	Cephalogram	0.449	< 0.001	Kitamura et al. [9]
		0.310	< 0.01	Sakakibara et al. [11]
		0.420	< 0.001	Yucel et al. [12]
TGL	Cephalogram	0.320	< 0.01	Yu et al. [10]
		0.213	< 0.05	Sakakibara et al. [11]
H-VL	Cephalogram	0.430	< 0.01	Yu et al. [10]
		0.425	< 0.001	Sakakibara et al. [11]
BMI	Other	0.310	< 0.001	Kitamura et al. [9]
		0.525		Sakakibara et al. [11]
MMP	Visual Exam.	0.316	< 0.001	Kitamura et al. [9]
Tonsil Size	Visual Exam.	0.212	0.005	Kitamura et al. [9]
Tongue Area in SP	2D MRI	0.441	< 0.01	Herrman et al. [19]
Tongue Circum.		0.446	< 0.01	Herrman et al. [19]
Neck Circum.		0.482	< 0.01	Hoffstein et al. [20]
Airway Vol.	3D MRI	0.098	0.58	Iida-Kondo et al. [13]

Our Approach in This Chapter

Snoring sounds and oropharyngeal soft tissues are directly or indirectly relate to the severity of SAS. Although many researchers still analyze these data, o approaches based on signal and image processing have not been considered ye The following sections are organized as follows.

The second section describes the differences among acoustic properti of snoring sounds produced by different respiratory routes; oral, nasal, ar oronasal inhalation. Since nasal congestion and open mouth during sleep a often regarded as risk factors of OSAS, recognizing such differences is a key identifying which part is easy to be corrupted when apnea occurs.

The third section demonstrates that morphological properties of tongue ar soft palate are related to the severity of OSAS. By using the results of our qua titative analysis of MRIs, you can recognize the typical shapes of these soft ti sues found in severe OSAS patients. Compared with a traditional cephalogran based method, our obtained knowledge is sufficiently simple and easy to understand. Moreover, the relation between snoring sounds and morphological properties of the soft tissues are discussed.

The fourth section focuses on some kind of unique snores; post-apneic snores. In general, these snores are said to be gasp-like sounds intrinsic to OSAS. But they have not been analyzed in detail, because their nonlinear and nonstationary properties make it difficult to properly calculate the spectra using traditional signal processing techniques. In this section, Hilbert-Huang transform (HHT) designed for analyzing this type of signals is applied to post-apneic snores and their nonlinearity and nonstationarity are quantitatively clarified based on the HHT spectra.

Finally, the last section is devoted to a conclusion and future works.

Acoustics of Oral, Nasal, and Oronasal Snoring Sounds

This section describes the differences among acoustic properties of snoring sounds produced by different respiratory routes; oral, nasal, and oronasal inhalation. Since nasal congestion and open mouth during sleep are often regarded as risk factors of OSAS, recognizing such differences is a key to identifying which part is easy to be corrupted when apnea occurs.

Relevance to Breath Routes during Sleep

Open mouth during sleep is often said to be related to loud snoring and OSAS, as it makes the lower jaw move backward and, in accordance with this, the surrounding soft tissues easily close the airway. Most loud snores are generated by vibrating the soft tissues under the large airflow with oral breath. Thus, oral appliances are sometimes used to stop loud snoring and sleep apnea.

In conventional studies, spectral properties of snoring sounds have been focused on to find out the intrinsic properties in OSAS patients. But spectral properties of snoring sounds have high diversity (as shown in Figures 2 to 4) reflected by breath routes and the corresponding non-simple mechanics of snore generation. It is thus necessary to clarify the concrete mechanism of such diversity so as to diagnose OSAS using the snoring sounds data, because even patients with the same severity do not necessarily have the same condition a each other. For example, airway obstruction may be caused by the enlargeme of the tongue and/or the soft palate. Moreover, the narrow airway caused b retrognathia or simple nasal congestion can possibly be considered. Naturall by using only snoring sounds data it is difficult to diagnose these conditio precisely, but these different conditions may reflect the spectral properties o snoring sounds. For example, retrognathia makes the jaw move backward an the airway comes to be narrow by tongue base corruption, leading to the snore generated by tongue base vibration. Nasal congestion makes the nasal rou closed, and thus oral breath generates loud snoring and the intrinsic propertie of snores with oral breath. Accordingly, recognizing the difference of snorin sounds among breath routes may possibly be useful for diagnosing OSAS co ditions.

In this section, the authors obtained simulated snoring sounds from 15 pe sons (including OSAS patients) and delineated the acoustic properties whe breathing orally, nasally, and oronasally. Simulated snoring sounds are not ac tual ones when sleeping, but Herzog, et al. [21], indicated that the acoust properties of them are equivalent to each other.

Data Acquisition and Analysis Method

A portable linear PCM (Pulse Code Modulation) sound recorder, Olympus LS 10, is used to record snoring sounds. Sampling frequency and quantization ra are set to 44.1 kHz and 16 bit respectively. Snoring sounds are recorded from 1 subjects and the recording time is about 30 seconds per person and per breat Before recording, the authors explained the objective of this study and obtaine the informed consent from all subjects.

The subjects are asked to simulate snoring by breathing deeply enough vibrate the soft palate in their throat. While producing oral snores, the subject nostrils are completely closed with their fingers, and on the other hand they a asked to let their mouth completely closed while producing nasal snores.

Such snoring, called *simulated snoring* in common, is not the one generate from a person during sleep, but it has traditionally been adopted in some medic studies [21] [22] [23] [24] [25].

Snore segments called *Episodes* are firstly extracted by hand from th recorded sleep sound (Figure 1). Since the acoustic properties of snoring soun

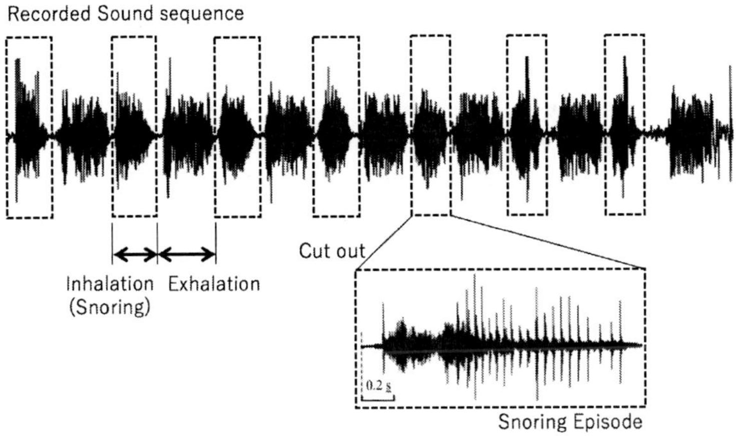

Figure 1. Manually extraction of snoring episodes from recorded sequential sounds.

are nonstationarily changing as time passes even in a snoring episode [26], the authors extracted short-time subsequences by sliding the window across the episode. This technique is commonly used in speech recognition. The windows prepared for extracting subsequences are 0.2 seconds in length and shifted 0.1 seconds. The extracted subsequence is expressed as $s(t)$, and in order to remove the effect of the microphone position, $s(t)$ is normalized to $E[s(t)] = 0$ and $E[s(t)^2] = 1$ where $E[\cdot]$ is an expectation operator. As a result, the authors can obtain 1,384 oral and 1,107 nasal and 1,229 oronasal subsequences from all subjects. Finally, spectral properties of the subsequences are calculated by Fast Fourier Transform (FFT) with Hanning window function.

Typical Properties of Three Breath Routes

Figures 2, 3 and 4 show typical examples of the FFT amplitude spectra of oral, nasal, and oronasal snoring sounds respectively. These properties are extremely different from each other, even in the time domain.

Nasal Snores

First of all, the authors can recognize that some nasal snores are clearly cycl waveforms and a few peaks in the frequency domain (Figure 2). Since one c the spectral peaks tends to be prominent, nasal snores mainly consist of a simp vibration (a single peak) with a few nonlinear effects (a few harmonic peaks Nasal snores do not necessarily show such simpler vibrations, but more comple or noisy waveforms as well, but almost all of the simpler waveforms are foun only in nasal snores.

The snore waveforms largely characterized by a single prominent peak i the frequency domain have also been reported in Beck and coworkers study [25 They called this type of snore a *simple waveform*. In our data, most simp waveforms are found in nasal snores.

Simple waveform snores are approximately explained by a linear vibratic system. According to Liistro's report [22], only uvula begins to vibrate, drive by inhalation airflow. This part gets caught in between oral and nasal brea route anatomically, but oral airway is completely closed with tongue when nas breathing. Only one side of the airflow is the driving force accordingly. There fore, the uvula is not only simply fluttering but with collision against the oth side of the airway wall (tongue). This nonlinear phenomenon depicts the vert cal asymmetry in the waveforms of the nasal snores and some harmonic peak in the frequency domain shown in Figure 2.

Oral Snores

Oral snores seem to be more complex than nasal ones from the viewpoint c both the waveforms and spectra. In Figure 3, the authors can find some period waveforms highly contaminated with noisy components in the range from 7(to 1.5 kHz, and that the fundamental frequency is relatively lower than th of nasal ones. In addition, the *formant*-like intensity peak commonly exists i every spectrum of the oral snores, whereas there are no such properties in nas snores.

Based on the Liistro's simple explanation [22], the sound source of or snore consists of both the soft palate and the tongue base, whereas nasal sno is only the vibration sound of the uvula, the tip of the soft palate. Accordingl lower fundamental frequency of oral snore is derived from the heavier ma

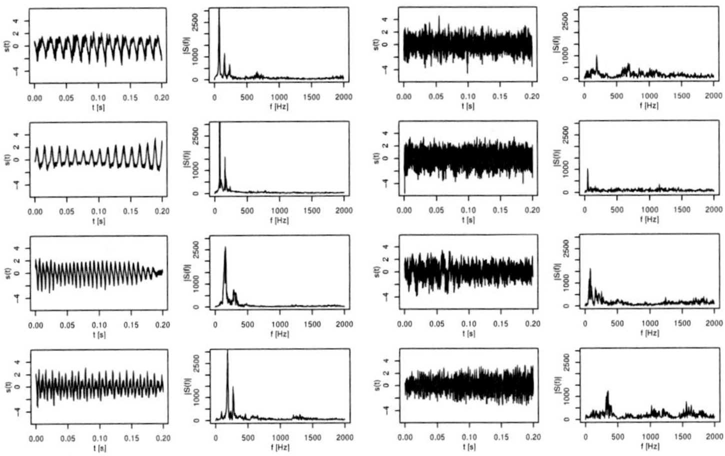

Figure 2. Waveforms and the amplitude spectra of periodic (left two columns) and non-periodic (right two columns) snoring sounds generated by nasal inhalation.

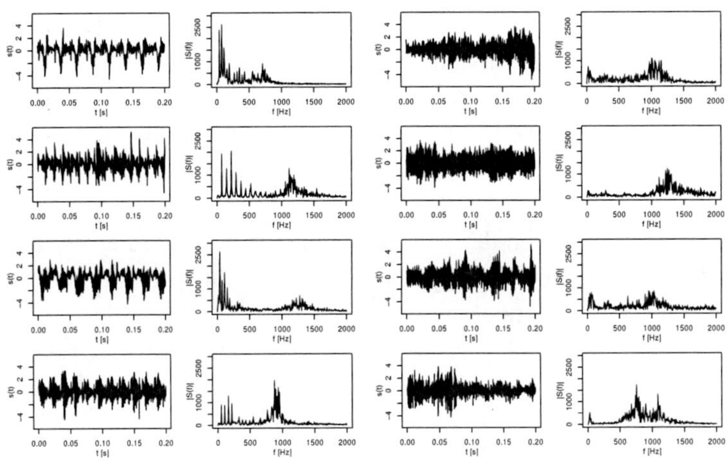

Figure 3. Waveforms and the amplitude spectra of periodic (left two columns) and non-periodic (right two columns) snoring sounds generated by oral inhalation.

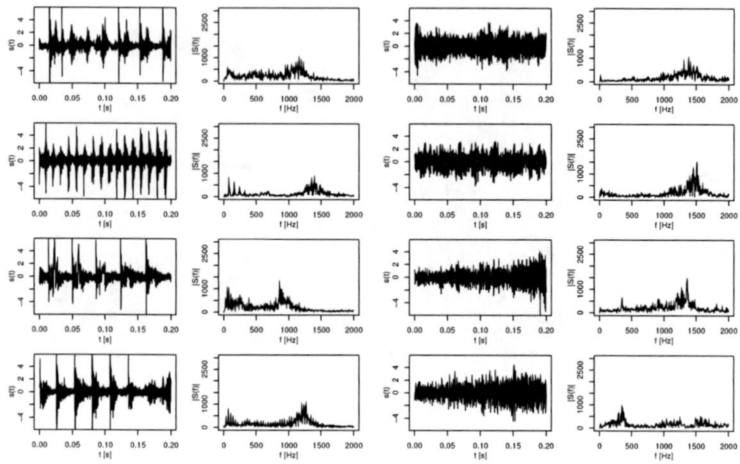

Figure 4. Waveforms and the amplitude spectra of periodic (left two column: and non-periodic (right two columns) snoring sounds generated by oronasal i halation

(whole soft palate including uvula) and the corresponding natural frequenc inversely proportional to the mass based on a mass-spring system. This is wh the oral snores have lower periodicity than nasal ones [25].

But, in some waveforms of oral snores, there is not any periodicity but th intensity peaks still remain (the second panel from the top in Figure 3). Thu it can be considered that the intensity peaks are more essential property of or snores than the periodicity. This may be attributed to a vibration and/or nois generated around the tongue base.

This intensity peak can be evaluated as a formant-like acoustic property ju like vowels. Also, the sound source may not be a linear/nonlinear vibratic because the spectrum does not consist of a single peak and its harmonic ones i the range from 700 to 1.5 kHz.

Many OSAS patients tend to breathe orally during sleep, and so these pro erties can be found more in OSAS patients.

Oronasal Snores

Besides, some of oronasal snores are similar to oral ones; the intensity peak in the range from 700 to 1.5 kHz is also found. But some of them are quite characteristic in Figure 4. These are composed of a series of impulses with lower frequency. Such properties have also been reported in conventional studies. Osborne et al. [27] insisted that this impulse-like features are derived from palatal snoring and Crest Factor Analysis is useful to discriminate the other snores. If this impulse-like waveforms are the result of palatal vibration, the vibration part would be rather slapping than vibrating.

It is difficult for subjects to precisely control their breathing both orally and nasally. The oronasal snores in our studies are not always precisely produced by oronasal breathing, but subjects' nostrils are not closed while snoring and they are asked to breathe through both as much as possible. Thus, some of oronasal snores are quite similar to oral ones.

Summary of This Section

There are two types of snoring sounds: periodic waveforms and noisy (non-periodic) waveforms. Oral and oronasal snores are periodic but includes noisy components as well. Their waveforms are relatively complex including not only single peak at the fundamental frequency but also their many harmonic ones. The noisy components are found in frequency domain ranging from 500 Hz to 1.5 kHz, although there are individual differences. They are similar to the formant peaks found in speech signals. Some researchers have pointed out that such formant-like features reflect the narrowed airway indicating precursors of OSAS [7] [8]. But, so far as the authors have investigated the acoustic properties, it seems not to be easy to conclude the relation between formant-like features and its relation to OSAS, because spectral properties in the same subject are quite various depending on the physiological conditions during sleep.

On the other hand, nasal snores tend not to be mixed with noisy components. Namely, either periodic vibrational or non-periodic noisy sound occurs. The fundamental frequency is slight higher than that of oral and oronasal snores. The waveform is relatively simple and in the frequency domain only a single spectral peak is dominant. This is caused by fluttering uvula without any non-linear phenomena [22].

MORPHOLOGICAL PROPERTIES OF OROPHARYNGEA SOFT TISSUES IN OSAS PATIENTS

This section demonstrates that morphological properties of tongue and other so tissues are related to the severity of OSAS. By using the results of our quantita tive analysis of MRIs, you can recognize the typical shapes of these soft tissue found in severe OSAS patients. Compared with a traditional cephalogram-base method, our obtained knowledge is sufficiently simple and easy to understan In the case of OSAS patients, over 80 % of SAS patients, the upper airway tenc to be narrower than benign persons even while awakening. By observing MI images, the authors can qualitatively recognize that enlargement of oropharyn geal soft tissues such as tonsils, soft palate, uvula, and tongue are main facto influencing narrowing of the upper airway.

This section mainly focused on the tongue morphology and indicates tha this property can potentially be a certain indicator to estimate the OSAS severit

Tablc 2. Photographing conditions of the sagittal and transverse planes i the upper airway MRIs

	T1-weighted Sagittal Plane	T1-weigted Transverse Plane
TE	12 ms	12 ms
TR	450 ms	518 ms
Field of View	256×256 mm^2	256×256 mm^2
Slice Thickness	4.5 mm	5 mm
Slice Gap	0.5 mm	1 mm
Num. of Slices	20	25
Matrix	205×205	205×205

Tongue Shapes of OSAS Patients

Traditionally, many researchers have focused on the relation between the vo ume or the area of the tongue and the severity. By observing the upper airwa

MR images of OSAS patients, the authors can also identify the importance of the tongue morphology.

The subjects are 82 male OSAS patients, who have received the medical treatment at Hakodate National Hospital. The upper airway MR images are obtained from all of them. The instrument is the InteraMaster R8 made by PHILIPS Co.Ltd., and the magnetic field strength is 1.5 T. The upper airway MR images analyzed here are composed of T1-weighted sagittal and transverse planes under the conditions shown in Table 2. While photographing, the subjects lie on their back in bed and their head is completely stabilized.

Compared among MR images obtained from mild, moderate, and severe OSAS patients, we can find that the tongue shapes of moderate or severe patients tend to be elongated diagonally along with the airway, whereas those of the mild patients are not elongated.

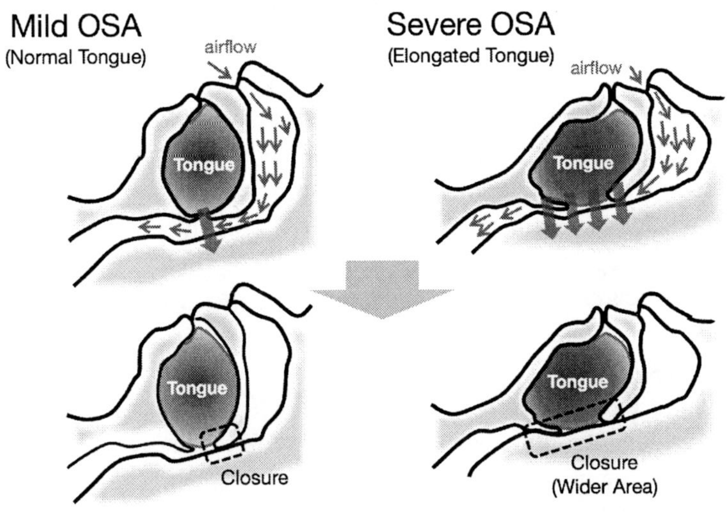

Figure 5. Tongue morphology and the relation to airway obstruction.

Why does such elongated tongue make the OSAS more severe? One answer may be considered by Bernoulli's effect based on the fluid mechanics. The airflow caused by inhalation decreases static pressure, and then the tongue base gravitates downwards and makes the airway narrower. This effect makes it easier to narrow the airway by increasing the airflow velocity, especially i the case of the narrowed airway or naturally narrow airway. In the case that th airway of the patients whose tongue is elongated, the wider area tends to grav itate downwards by Bernoulli's effect, and therefore airway obstruction woul become more serious. On the other hand, non-elongated tongue is not so eas ily collapsed. Even if collapsed, the airway may be closed during short-tim (Figure 5).

Image-Based Analysis of Tongue Morphology

In this subsection, the authors quantitatively evaluate the tongue morpholog found in severe OSAS patients described in the previous subsection. In order t evaluate the morphological features of the tongue region in the sagittal plane, is necessary to perform the segmentation of the tongue region. In convention studies, segmentation of many organs has been performed in various algorithm such as brain [28], liver [29], and blood vessels [30] [31]. But no methods of th tongue region segmentation have been proposed. Since conventional methoc for the other organs are based on the own characteristics, they cannot necessaril be applied to the tongue segmentation. Thus, the authors considered it difficu to develop an automation technique for the tongue region segmentation and fo now decided to extract the tongue region manually one by one on the OsiriX, medical image processing software.

The center of gravity of the whole extracted tongue region is firstly calcu lated. From this point, straight lines are radially extended at the fixed angul intervals of $\theta = \pi/48$ radian, and the radius L_i $(i = 1, 2, \cdots, 96)$ from th center to the circumference of the tongue region is estimated (Figure 6). Sinc the patients lie on the bed while photographing, vertical direction in the imag indicates the bed surface and is defined as zero radian. In addition, $L_i(n)$ defined as ith length of nth subject. Such feature extraction method has widel been used in many pattern recognition applications [32].

The quantified morphological features estimated from the upper airwa MRIs are evaluated by calculating the correlation coefficient, R, (Pearson's co relation) with Apnea/Hypopnea Index (AHI). Let $X(n)$ be one of the morpho logical features estimated from the nth subject, and AHI(n) is the value of AH estimated from PSG screening of the nth subject. The correlation coefficien

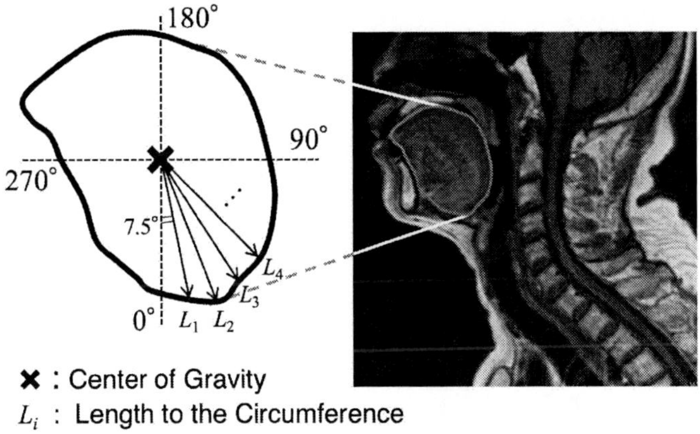

Figure 6. Quantitative evaluation of the tongue morphology in sagittal MR image.

R, is calculated by

$$R = \frac{\sum_{n=1}^{N}(\mathrm{AHI}(n) - \overline{\mathrm{AHI}})(X(n) - \overline{X})}{\sqrt{\sum_{n=1}^{N}(\mathrm{AHI}(n) - \overline{\mathrm{AHI}})^2}\sqrt{\sum_{n=1}^{N}(X(n) - \overline{X})^2}}, \tag{1}$$

where $\overline{X}$ and $\overline{\mathrm{AHI}}$ are, respectively, calculated by

$$\overline{X} = \frac{1}{N}\sum_{n=1}^{N} X(n), \tag{2}$$

$$\overline{\mathrm{AHI}} = \frac{1}{N}\sum_{n=1}^{N} \mathrm{AHI}(n), \tag{3}$$

where N is the number of subjects ($N = 82$).

Figure 7 shows the correlation coefficients of $L_1 - L_{96}$ with AHI. The correlation value is over 0.5 if $i = 5, \cdots, 9$ and $i = 48, 49, \cdots, 56$. Each of these directions are, respectively, called A ($i = 5, 6, \cdots, 9$) and B ($i = 48, 49, \cdots, 56$). In the region A, the maximum correlation is $R = 0.578$ ($p < 0.001$) when

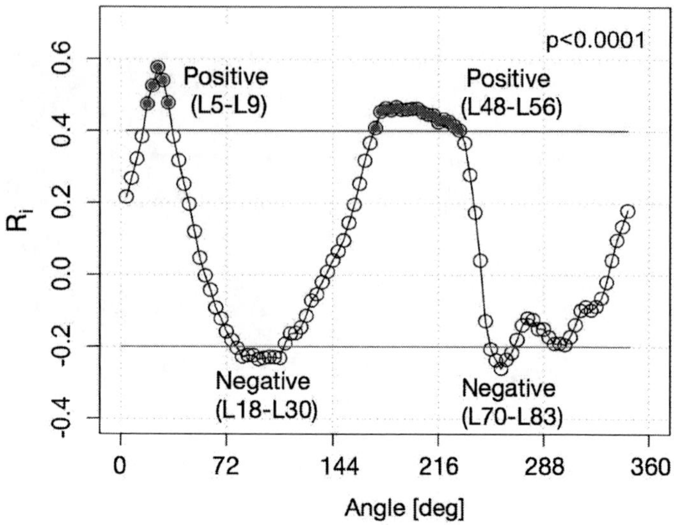

Figure 7. Correlation coefficient between L_i and the OSAS severity.

$i = 7$, while in the region B the maximum correlation is $R = 0.482$ ($p < 0.00$ when $i = 51$. Moreover, the directions of $i = 18, \cdots, 30$ and its point symm try $i = 70, \cdots, 83$ have negative correlation to the severity (minimum value -0.275 with $p < 0.001$).

According to the results, the morphological property of the tongue in seve OSAS patients is the diagonally elongation (Figure 8), whose direction forms a angle of 26.25 degree from the vertical to the lower-right (L_7). This result shov the correctness of our qualitative discussion. But the physical mechanism of th airway obstruction caused by the tongue elongation should be further verifie with physical modeling or computer simulation.

In addition, since cephalometry does not provide any information of th tongue elongation, our method has an advantage in comparison with conve tional methods. Naturally, it is difficult to simply compare these results wi each other, because the number of subjects and subjects' AHI are differe among these reports. But, so far as Table 1 or 3 indicates, the authors can sa that our result is far better than the other features and significant as well.

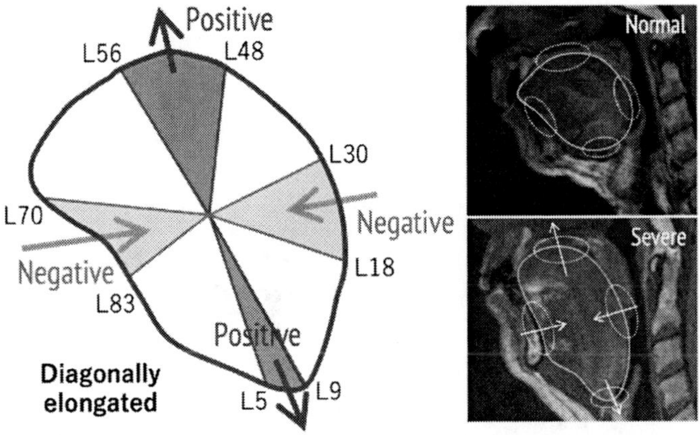

Figure 8. The tongue shape correlated with the severity of OSAS.

Some Exception Examples

Diagonally elongation of the tongue is an important property of severe OSAS patients, but there are some exceptions because the OSAS is caused by multiple factors. Figure 9 shows some exceptions, the each panel in which the tongue is not elongated at all and the airway is not so narrowed as well.

But the subject A, the left panel in Figure 9, is a severe OSAS patient (AHI = 39). His apnea is accompanied by depression, and he took some psychotropic medications. Traditionally, it has been known that taking psychotropic medications can be a worsening factor for SAS [33] and in such cases it is difficult to detect OSAS only using the sagittal tongue morphology.

Next, in the center panel in Figure 9, the subject B has a sufficient airway and his tongue is not elongated. So far as our image-based criterion is applied, he may not be recognized as a severe patient. But this patient is a severe OSAS patient (AHI = 41) with lower 74 % of SpO2. He has allergic rhinitis and the corresponding nasal closure. Nasal closure is also known to be a risk factor for OSAS [34]. This type of OSAS patient cannot be detected using our method.

In the subject C in Figure 9, although back of the tongue looks slightly raised, tongue is not so diagonally elongated. The soft palate is tick, but the airway seems to be sufficiently wide. His AHI is 38.4, a severe patient. I this case, the authors recognized from the transverse plane that the tonsils a enlarged. The airway obstruction of this patient is not caused by the tongu elongation, but by the tonsil enlargement. Also, this is not observed in a sagitt plane.

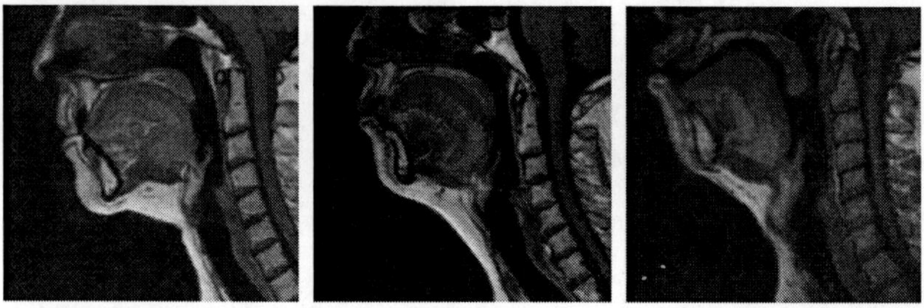

Figure 9. Severe OSAS patients who cannot be detected using tongue morpho ogy.

Other Soft Tissues

Tonsil enlargement is not recognized in a sagittal plane, but in a transverse plan Even if the tongue morphology is not elongated, some patients have a seve OSAS caused by the enlargement of other soft tissues such as tonsils and/or so palate, which leads to the airway obstruction.

Thus, the authors have evaluated the correlation between the cross section area of the narrowest point in the upper airway and the severity of OSAS (Fi ure 10). As as result, the correlation coefficient is -0.354. This means that th smaller cross sectional area makes OSAS more severe. Compared with Table this correlation is largely equivalent to the one estimated from skull properti using cephalogram in conventional studies [10] [11]. Although the tongue mo phology is more correlated with the severity, the enlargement of the soft pala or tonsils is also correlated to the severity.

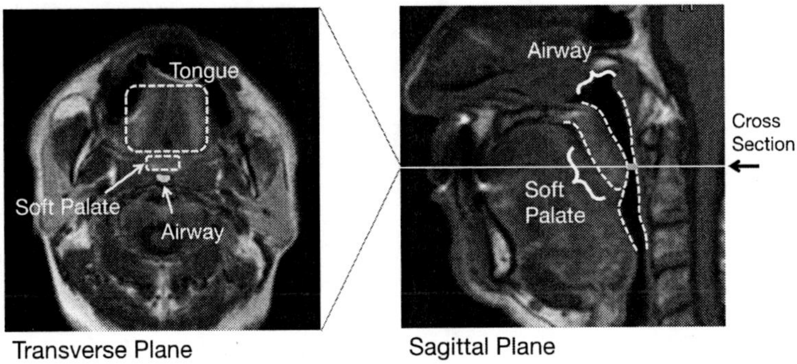

Figure 10. Evaluation of the cross sectional area around the soft palate and tonsils.

Summary of This Section

Table 3 shows some morphological properties that lead to higher correlation with AHI. By using a sagittal MR images, it is possible that the severity of OSAS can largely be recognized. Our quantitative evaluation of the tongue morphology shows that the length at 26.25 degree from the lower vertical line is most correlated to the OSAS severity, namely, the tongue is diagonally elongated. The correlation coefficient between the length of this direction and the severity becomes nearly 0.6. Compared with other traditional properties (Tables 1 and 3), this is the highest correlation with the severity and thus our image-based criterion is useful for detecting severe OSAS.

However, similar to the other image-based method, our criterion is not a decisive method. In the previous section, the authors introduced some exceptions which cannot be recognized using tongue morphology. In addition, the deepness of sleep (the first night effect), the muscle relaxation, and the effect of pills for various illness simultaneously suffered are also considered risk factors. Although PSG is known to be a gold standard screening, the authors cannot completely avoid the first night effect. Accordingly, our obtained knowledge would be a useful image-based method as an approach to the recognition of severe OSAS different from a traditional PSG.

Table 3. Correlation between AHI and morphologic properties in our studies

Feature	Method	Corr. Coef.	p-value
L_7	Sagittal MRI	0.578	< 0.001
L_{51}	Sagittal MRI	0.482	< 0.001
cross sectional area	Transverse MRI	-0.354	0.02

NONLINEAR AND NONSTATIONARY PROPERTIES OF POST-APENIC SNORES

We focus on some kinds of unique snores; post-apneic snores. In this sectio we basically review our paper [35]. In general, these snores are said to be gas like sounds intrinsic to Obstructive sleep apnea syndrome (OSAS) and the are some researches tried to discover intrinsic properties of the snoring soun in OSAS patients discussed in the subsection of "Evaluation of Soft Tissues i Conventional Studies". However, these conventional results are different fro each other. Moreover, since their nonlinear and nonstationary properties mak it difficult to properly calculate the spectra using traditional signal processin techniques, such as FFT and Linear Predictive Coding (LPC).

In this section, Hilbert-Huang Transform (HHT) [36], which is designed f analyzing nonlinear and nonstationary signals, is adopted to generate a tim frequency map of post-apneic snores and the temporal variation in the spe tral density is quantitatively evaluated using the averaged Kullback-Leibler d vergence. Then we discusses the nonlinear and nonstationarity of post-apne snores revealed by our results, and the relevant physiological mechanism. The are some researches on applications of HHT for the analysis of oronasal airwa pressure signals [37] [38], but to the best of our knowledge, no prior studi exist that apply HHT to such snoring sounds.

Strategy

The overview of our strategy used in this section is shown in Figure 11.

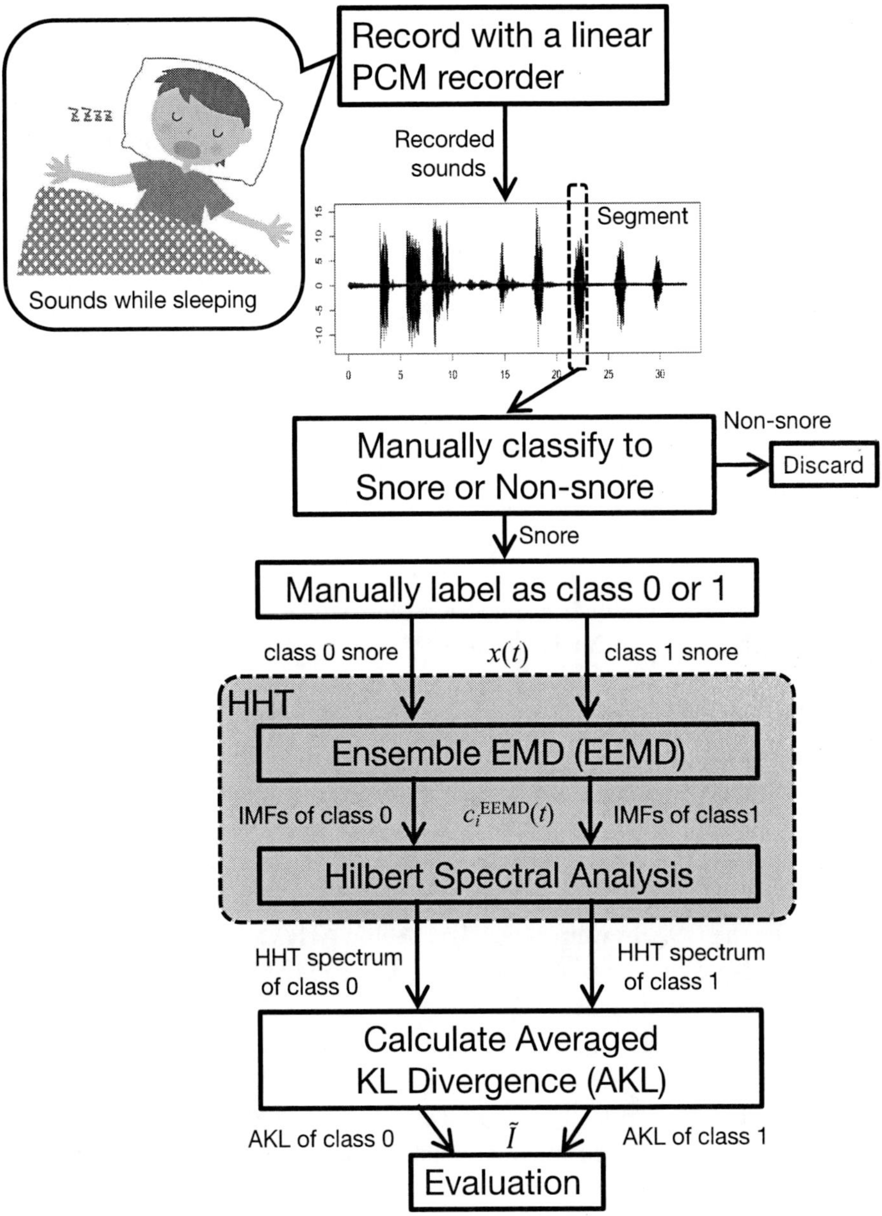

Figure 11. Strategy of the analysis.

Data Collection, Calculation of Severity and Labelling of Snores

We studied seven patients with severe OSAS who were outpatients at the slee clinic at Hakodate National Hospital and required hospitalization-based test Table 4 lists the gender, age, and OSAS severity, of the subjects. While patien underwent polysomnography (PSG) in the hospital, their snores were recorde using a bedside sound recording device. The recording device used was th Olympus LS-11 linear PCM recorder. The sampling rate was 44.1 kHz, an the audio bit depth was 16. No data compression was performed and the m crophone was not oriented in any specific direction. The external micropho used was the Olympus ME30W, which was fixed to a pillar at the head-end the bed. Recording was continuous from the time the patient went to bed u til they got up the following morning, generating approximately 7-10 hours recording time.

The continuous recordings over 7-10 hours throughout the night are als contained by a variety of sounds other than the snores that would be subjecte to analysis, such as talking, coughing, doors opening and closing, breathi during sleep, talking during sleep, the sound of car engines, ambulance siren and the sound of blankets during sleep. The snore signals that were subje to the conducted analyses were manually extracted from these. Moreover, the case that snore and other sounds are recorded at the same time, such sou segments are classified to non-snore shown in Figure 11, namely, excluded fro the analysis targets.

Based on the American Academy of Sleep Medicine (AASM) definitio of apnea, hypopnea, and OSAS, and the apnea/hypopnea index (AHI; avera frequency of apnea or hypopnea over 1 hour of sleep), will be used to dete mine the OSAS severity. For the specific AHI values, data were used that we calculated from the subjects' PSG data acquired by clinical technologists at th Hakodate National Hospital.

Furthermore, while referring to PSG results, the obtained snore data we divided into two classes. The first contained the post-apneic snores, and th second all other data. These classes were labeled as "class 0" and "class 1 respectively. Comparing the number of snore data for class 0 and class 1, cla 0 snores were approximately 20, whereas class 1 snores were several hundre Therefore, 50 datasets were randomly extracted from the data labeled as cla 1 for data analyses. Table 4 shows the class 0 and class 1 data obtained

Table 4. The number of snoring sounds classified in accordance to class 0 and class 1 in all subjects. The "class 0" contains the post-apneic snores, and "class 1" is all other data. This table is made based on the data of Table 1 in [35]

Subject	Gender	Age	AHI	# of class 0	# of class 1
A	Male	65	47.4	20	50
B	Male	52	56.2	20	50
C	Male	21	42.4	8	50
D	Female	75	31.0	10	50
E	Male	46	33.5	12	50
F	Female	62	34.7	9	50
G	Male	74	40.1	0	50
Average	–	56.4	40.8	11.3	50.0

described above. Occurrence of snores was very rare for subject G compared to other subjects, while class 0 snores were absent.

Hilbert-Huang Transform

The Hilbert-Huang transform (HHT) is a time-frequency analysis method [36], which is constructed under the aim to manipulate non-stationary and/or non-linear system. The HHT is based on a signal analysis by the Hilbert transform. We describe the concept of the signal analysis by the Hilbert transform and its difficulty to be applied to real-world signals, and then explain how the HHT overcomes the difficulty.

Note that the data $s(t)$ are continuous time signals, and are discretized at discrete time intervals, $t_n = n\Delta t$, where $n = 0, 1, \cdots, N-1$, N is the number of data points, and Δt is the sampling interval. However, the subscription n is abbreviated when no confusion likely arise.

Letting $\hat{s}(t)$ be the Hilbert transform of a signal $s(t)$, it is defined by

$$\hat{s}(t) = \frac{1}{\pi} \mathrm{PV} \int \mathrm{d}t' \, \frac{s(t')}{t - t'}, \tag{4}$$

where PV denotes the Cauchy principal value. The complex signal $z(t)$, whic is defined by $z(t) = s(t) + \mathrm{i}\hat{s}(t)$, can be represented by the exponential form:

$$z(t) = a(t)\mathrm{e}^{\mathrm{i}\phi(t)}\,, \qquad (5)$$

where $a(t)$ and $\phi(t)$ are defined by

$$a(t) = \sqrt{s(t)^2 + \hat{s}(t)^2}\,, \qquad (6)$$

$$\phi(t) = \arctan\left(\frac{\hat{s}(t)}{s(t)}\right). \qquad (7)$$

Therefore,

$$s(t) = a(t)\cos\phi(t), \qquad (8)$$

is established. Only when the signal $s(t)$ is monochromatic over short perio of time, $z(t)$ is an analytic signal of $s(t)$, in other words, the Fourier compo nents of $z(t)$ are the same as $s(t)$ in the positive frequency range, and zero the negative frequency range [39], and then $a(t) = \mathrm{IA}(t)$ and $\phi(t) = \mathrm{IP}($ are called instantaneous amplitude (IA) and instantaneous phase (IP) of $s(t$ respectively. The monochromaticity of $s(t)$ over short periods of time mear that $\mathrm{IA}(t)$ has only lower frequency components than $\cos\mathrm{IP}(t)$, or $\mathrm{IA}(t)$ ar $\cos\mathrm{IP}(t)$ are the modulator and the carrier of the signal $s(t)$, respectively. that case, the local mean $m(t)$ of $s(t)$, which is defined by

$$m(t) = \frac{u(t) + l(t)}{2}\,, \qquad (9)$$

where $u(t)$ and $l(t)$ are the upper and lower envelopes of $s(t)$, respectively, zero at any point. We call this feature *zero-mean*. An instantaneous frequenc (IF) of $s(t)$ is defined by

$$\mathrm{IF}(t) = \frac{1}{2\pi}\frac{\mathrm{dIP}(t)}{\mathrm{d}t}\,. \qquad (10)$$

This analysis to estimate the IA and IF from a signal is called the Hilbert spe tral analysis (HSA). The HSA has an advantage of higher resolution than th other time-frequency analysis such as the short-time Fourier transform (STF and the Wavelet transform. However, it cannot be applied to most real-wor signals, because they are basically composites of some components and are not monochromatic. Huang et al. [36] overcame the difficulty by combining a mode decomposition part with the HSA, and the method of combination of them is the HHT.

Huang et al. developed a method to decompose an input data $x(t)$ into zero-mean components and a non-oscillatory component. They named the method empirical mode decomposition (EMD) and also named the decomposed zero-mean components intrinsic mode functions (IMFs) of the input data. Algorithm 1 shows the procedure of the EMD, where $c_i(t)$ and $r(t)$ are the ith IMF and a non-oscillatory component of $x(t)$, respectively. Figure 12 also shows a schematic overview of the EMD algorithm. Let me consider the EMD of an input data $x(t)$ shown in Figure 12(a). The first step is forming the upper envelope $u_{i,j}(t)$ and the lower envelope $l_{i,j}(t)$, connecting the maxima and the minima of the data by cubic splines (Figure 12(b)). Then, the mean $m_{i,j}(t)$ of these envelope is subtracted from the input data to obtain the residual $x_{i,(j+1)}$ (Figure 12(c)). When the mean $m_{i,j}(t)$ becomes approximately zero after several iterations, $x_{i,j}$ is adopted as the IMF $c_i(t)$, since it can be considered to be zero-mean (Figure 12(d)). This criteria ϵ_{e} is a parameter of the EMD [36] [40]. After all oscillatory components are extracted, the residual $r(t)$ is a non-oscillatory component of $x(t)$. Figure 13 shows the schematic result of EMD, with the input $x(t)$ decomposed into four IMFs and residual. Letting N_{IMF} be the number of IMFs of $x(t)$, $x(t)$ is recovered by

$$x(t) = \sum_{i=1}^{N_{\mathrm{IMF}}} c_i(t) + r(t)\,. \tag{11}$$

IMFs, $c_1(t)$, $c_2(t)$, $\ldots$, $c_{N_{\mathrm{IMF}}}(t)$, are in order from the highest to the lowest frequency components. After the above decomposition, the IA and IP of each IMF can be estimated by the HSA. Consequently, letting $\mathrm{IA}_i(t)$, $\mathrm{IP}_i(t)$ and $\mathrm{IF}_i(t)$ be the IA, IP and IF of ith IMF, the data can be expressed as

$$x(t) = \sum_{i=1}^{N_{\mathrm{IMF}}} \mathrm{IA}_i(t) \cos \mathrm{IP}_i(t) + r(t)\,, \tag{12}$$

$$\mathrm{IF}_i(t) = \frac{1}{2\pi} \frac{\mathrm{dIP}_i(t)}{\mathrm{d}t}\,. \tag{13}$$

Note that $\mathrm{IF}_i(t)$, which is defined as a function of time, has a different mear ing than the meaning of a Fourier frequency, which is defined as a consta frequency. Since $\mathrm{IF}_i(t)$ is a continuous function, fundamental frequency moc ulation can also be achieved.

Algorithm 1 Empirical mode decomposition

$i = 1$, $x_1(t) = x(t)$.
while $x_i(t)$ contains oscillatory components **do**
    $j = 1$, $x_{i,1}(t) = x_i(t)$
    while the local mean of $x_{i,j}(t)$ is not zero **do**
        $u_{i,j}(t) =$ (the upper envelope of $x_{i,j}(t)$).
        $l_{i,j}(t) =$ (the lower envelope of $x_{i,j}(t)$).
        $m_{i,j}(t) = (u_{i,j}(t) + l_{i,j}(t))/2$.
        $x_{i,(j+1)}(t) = x_{i,j}(t) - m_{i,j}(t)$.
        $j = j + 1$
    end while
    $c_i(t) = x_{i,j}(t)$
    $x_{i+1}(t) = x_i(t) - c_i(t)$.
    $i = i + 1$.
end while
$r(t) = x_i(t)$

It is known that EMD frequently observes the phenomena associated wit a number of frequency components intermingling in one IMF (mode mixing or the components of the same frequency band that are being dispersed ov multiple IMFs (mode splitting) [41]. In this research, we used the ensen ble EMD (EEMD) as the mode decomposition method. The EEMD is a improved method of EMD proposed by Wu and Huang [41]. In the begi ning of the EEMD, N_e white (Gaussian) noises $\{w^{(m)}(t)\}$ with the standar deviation being σ_e are created, and then the IMFs of the noise-added da

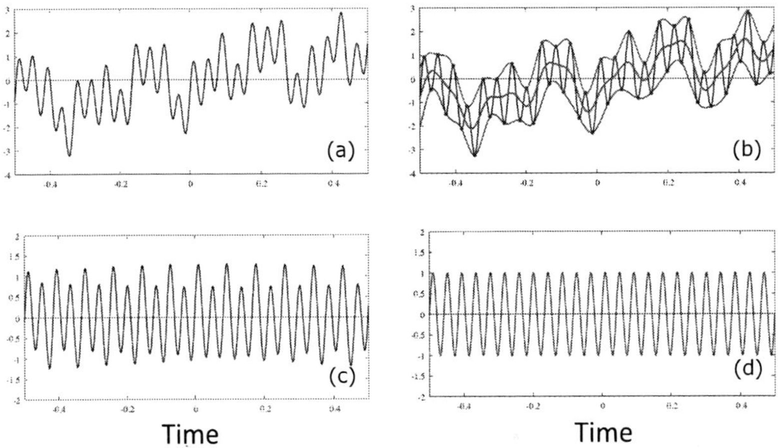

Figure 12. Schematic example of EMD process.

$x^{(m)}(t) = x(t) + w^{(m)}(t)$ are calculated by the EMD:

$$x^{(m)}(t) = x(t) + w^{(m)}(t) \tag{14}$$

$$= \sum_{i=1}^{N_{\mathrm{IMF}}} c_i^{(m)}(t) + r^{(m)}. \tag{15}$$

The IMFs of an input data $x(t)$ are estimated as the mean of the corresponding IMFs of $\{x^{(m)}(t)\}$:

$$c_i^{\mathrm{EEMD}}(t) = \frac{1}{N_{\mathrm{e}}} \sum_{m=1}^{N_{\mathrm{e}}} c_i^{(m)}(t). \tag{16}$$

The EEMD has three parameters $(\epsilon_{\mathrm{e}}, \sigma_{\mathrm{e}}, N_{\mathrm{e}})$. ϵ_{e} is a convergence-condition constant, σ_{e} is a standard deviation of added white noise, and N_{e} is the number of repeats. These parameters must be set appropriately, and the technique to achieve this has been discussed previously [42]. Here, we chose $\epsilon_{\mathrm{e}} = 10^{-1}, 10^{-2}, 10^{-3}, 10^{-4}, 10^{-5}$. The decomposition sometimes gets worse with more rigid criterion, or with small value of ϵ_{e}. It is because mode mixing

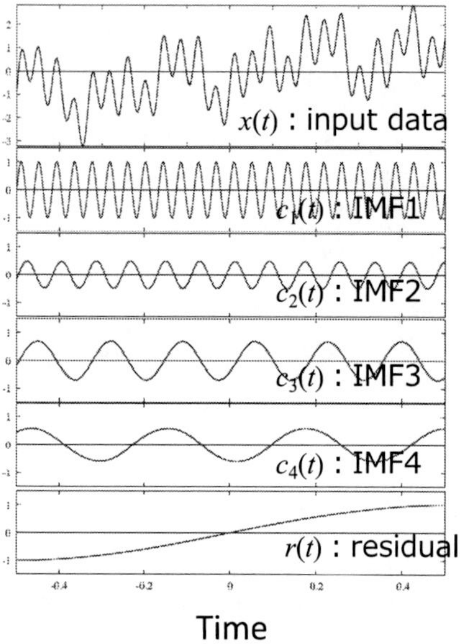

Figure 13. Schematic example of EMD result.

and/or mode splitting occur to a certain extent. We confirmed that the value o $\epsilon_{\mathrm{e}} = 10^{-3}$ was better than other values. For the EEMD, we used the standa deviation of the added white (Gaussian) noise of $\sigma_{\mathrm{e}} = 10^{-5}, 10^{-6}, 10^{-7}$. A though the dependence of the decomposition on σ_{e} was rather weak, the small value of σ_{e} was better. We chose the size of the ensemble to be $N_{\mathrm{e}} = 200$. W tried other values of N_{e}, and we verified that the results change little even wi $N_{\mathrm{e}} > 100$ but that $N_{\mathrm{e}} \sim 50$ was too small. Thus, in remaining of this pape we used the following parameter set: $\epsilon_{\mathrm{e}} = 10^{-3}$, $N_{\mathrm{e}} = 200, \sigma_{\mathrm{e}} = 10^{-7}$. Mo details of EEMD is shown in [40,41].

HSA is applied to each obtained IMF $c_i^{\mathrm{EEMD}}(t)$ shown in Eq.(16). Throug this process, instantaneous time-amplitude and time-frequency trajectories ca be extracted (Figure 14, left upper side). The distribution of time, frequenc and amplitude is collective referred to as the HHT spectrum or HHT map.

The complexity of HHT is due in large to EEMD part, depending on the si

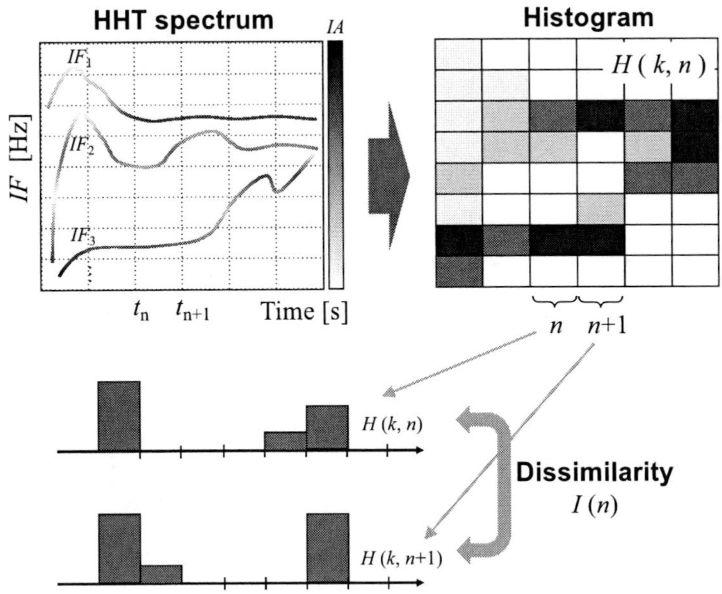

Figure 14. Dissimilarity between $H(k, n)$ and $H(k, n + 1)$ eliminated from the HHT Spectrum.

of the ensemble N_e. On the other hand, the Hilbert transforms can be performed: $2N_{\text{IMF}} \times N \log N$. This computational cost is smaller than that of EEMD. If we set $N_e = 200$, $N_{\text{IMF}} = 8$, $N = 44100$ (1 sec data), we can analyze within a few ten seconds by using one core of the modern cluster (CPU: Xeon E5-2667v4 (3.2GHz/8core 25MB) $\times$ 2, memory: 128GB (8 GB/core)).

Evaluation Method of Nonstationarity through HHT Spectrum

Figure 14 shows the schematic of evaluation method. Coarse graining is calculated using the HHT spectrum over a brief period of time. Then the result is represented in a histogram. The amount of change associated with the time variation in this histogram is quantified.

The discrete HHT spectrum is represented with $S'(k, n)$. However, the notation used is $k = 0, 1, 2, \cdots, 9$ and $n = 0, 1, 2, \cdots, N - 1$. Since N depends on the duration of the snore, it varies depending on the data. $S'(k,n)$ is an inte grated value for $\mathrm{IA}(\mathrm{IF},t)$ in the ranges of $\mathrm{IF} = \mathrm{IF}_k - \mathrm{IF}_{k+1}$, and $t = t_n - t_{n+}$

$$S'(k,n) = \int_{t_n}^{t_{n+1}} \int_{\mathrm{IF}_k}^{\mathrm{IF}_{k+1}} \mathrm{IA}(\mathrm{IF},t) d\mathrm{IF}\, dt\,, \quad (1$$

where $\mathrm{IF}_k = k \cdot \mathrm{DIF}$, $t_n = n \cdot D_t$, DIF $= 200$ Hz and $D_t = 750\Delta t$ secon (Δt is the sampling interval). These values are obtained empirically by choo ing various values for DIF and D_t. We then used the Kullback-Leibler (KL divergence as a measure of dissimilarity of $S'(\forall k,n)$ and $S'(\forall k,n+1)$ in and $n+1$. In other words, given $H(k,n) = S'(k,n)/\sum_k S'(k,n)$,

$$I(n) = \sum_{k=0}^{9} H(k,n) \log \frac{H(k,n)}{H(k,n+1)}\,, \quad (1$$

is obtained. A useful technique has been traditionally used that considers th power spectrum as a probability density through normalization, and represen the inter-spectral dissimilarity using KL divergence [43] [44].

After calculating $I(n)$ for $n = 0,1,2,\cdots,N-2$ its mean value $\tilde{I}$ is eval ated as the nonstationarity of snores:

$$\tilde{I} = \frac{1}{N-1} \sum_{n=0}^{N-2} I(n)\,. \quad (1$$

The mean KL divergence $\tilde{I}$ is calculated for each subject, and nonstationari differences for classes 0 and 1 are verified. For instance, if for all k, $H(k,n)$ ar $H(k,n+1)$ are exactly the same (if stationarity exists), then $I(n) = 0$ becau $H(k,n)/H(k,n+1) = 1$. The elicited value is the minimum value. Th can be interpreted as an increasing nonstationarity (i.e. the difference betwe neighboring spectra is increasing) with $I(n)$ attaining larger values.

Results and Discussion

Figure 15(a) and (b) illustrate typical time-series data (Signal) and intrins mode functions (IMF1-6) for class 0 and class 1 snores, respectively. In th case, the data is decomposed into 8 IMFs, but those only from IMF1 to IMI

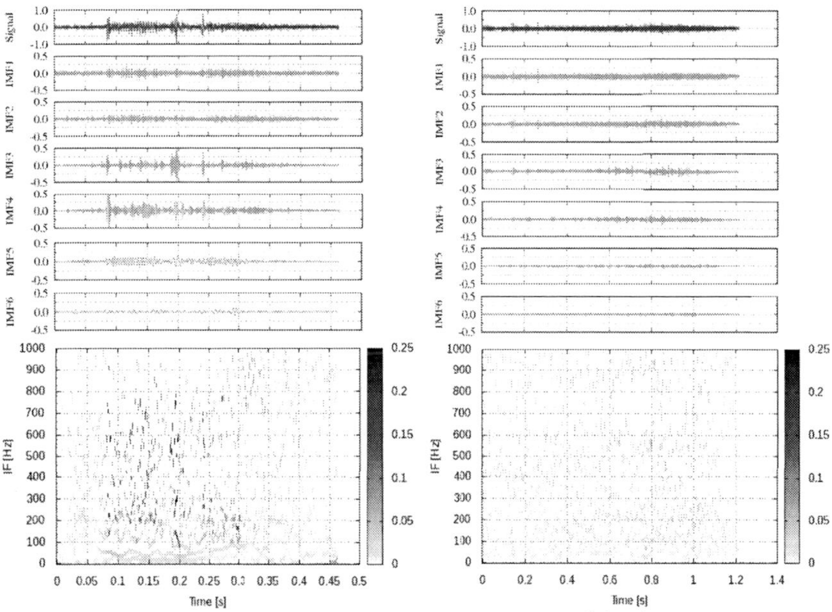

(a) class 0 (b) class 1

Figure 15. An example of a waveform (Signal), the estimated intrinsic mode functions (IMF1-6) and HHT spectrum. (a) Results for the snoring sounds that belong to class 0 and (b) Results for the snoring sounds that belong to class 0. IMF7-8 were calculated but we did not show them in the figures of IMF since IMF7-8 were almost monochromatic.

are plotted, since it is clear that no useful information is included in IMF7 and IMF8 i.e. IMF7 and IMF8 is almost monochromatic. HTT spectrums obtained from the intrinsic mode functions for class 0 and class 1 snores are also shown.

What can be confirmed from the waveforms of the time-series data (Signal) is that nonstationarity is higher for class 0 than for class 1 waveforms, and that waveform features change within a brief period of time. Although amplitude is variable for class 1 waveforms, no significant waveform changes are seen overall. However, for class 0 waveforms, altered waveform features can be confirmed at 0.08 seconds, within the ranges of 0.18-0.20 seconds, and at 0.24

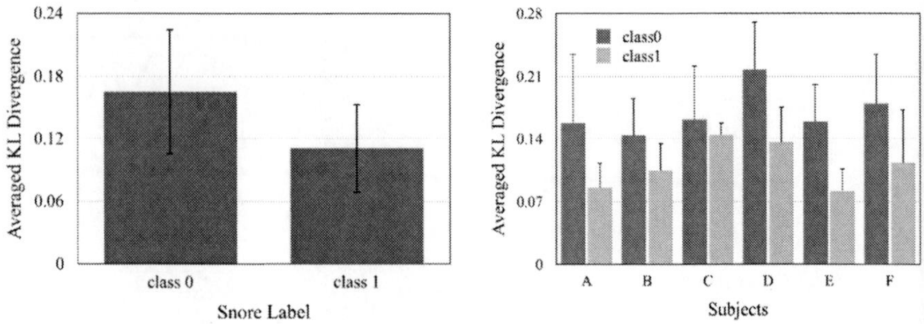

(a) (b)

Figure 16. Results of averaged KL divergence of class 0 and class 1. (a) Resu for all subjects using HHT ($p < 10^{-6}$) and (b) Intra-subject variability of th averaged KL divergence.

seconds. Features reflecting this type of nonstationarity can also be clearly see in IMF3 and IMF4. Whereas class 0 IMFs are divided into multiple, nonstatio ary IMFs, which are localized in terms of time, class 1 IMFs have no tempor locality from the onset to the end of the episode. This is also evident fro the HTT spectrum in the bottom of Figure 15(a) and (b). In the case of cla 0, the instantaneous frequency on the vertical axis shows nonstationary var ability, whereas this phenomenon is not observed for class 1. Although som differences were noted, these class 0 and class 1 characteristics were common evidenced in the waveforms acquired from all subjects.

By using averaged KL divergence, a quantitative evaluation was performe for all subjects in relation to the results elicited from class 0 snores (post-apne snores) that have nonstationarity.

Figure 16(a) shows the averages and standard deviations of $\tilde{I}$ for class 0 an for class 1 calculated from all subjects' data. Since $p < 10^{-6}$, a significa statistical difference was observed for class 0 and class 1. These results sho that the averaged KL divergence is higher for class 0 than for class 1 snore Therefore, nonstationarity is objectively shown to be higher for class 0.

Figure 16(b) shows the averages and standard deviations of $\tilde{I}$ calculated f class 0 and class 1 for each subject. Results show that even when the valu of $\tilde{I}$ belong in the same class 0, they vary substantially between subjects. For example, the value for class 0 for subject B is almost the same as those for class 1 for subject C and D. However, by focusing on the same subject, there is a tendency that the value of $\tilde{I}$ for class 0 is relatively higher than that for class 1. Furthermore, since $p < 0.05$ for all subjects, it can be concluded that there is a significant statistical difference between the results from class 0 and class 1.

Here, we discusses the nonstationarity of post-apneic snores revealed by our results, and the relevant physiological mechanism. The main reason for the occurrence of the snoring sounds is the vibration of soft oral tissues, but the dynamics are complex. Beck et al. have indicated that OSAS patients have narrower airways than healthy persons. For this reason, when the airway walls vibrate, they impact on each other leading to a temporary airway obstruction, which differs from the simple fluttering documented in the snoring of healthy persons [25]. Conversely, the airflow associated with the intake phase while the airway is in an opened state, can be said to be normal throughout. This can also be seen in the IMF in Figure 15(a). Additionally, the difference between class 0 and class 1 in the histograms in Figure 16(a) is believed to be the manifestation of the nonstationary property of the airflow when apnea reverts to breathing.

The results, shown in Figure 16(b), also revealed that there are substantial individual differences in regard to the nonstationarity of this type of post-apneic snores. These are believed to be owing to individual differences in various aspects, such as the morphological features of the obstruction site and the state of muscular relaxation. For instance, the most important factor in severe OSAS is a swollen soft palate or tongue, and these sites form an important source of snoring sounds, and display different acoustic properties. Conversely, there are also cases where these areas do not display much swelling, but where severe OSAS occurs owing to other causes, including skeletal characteristics, or muscle relaxation [45]. The present study focused on the snores of severe OSAS patients, but pathologies varied, and these types of differences are believed to be the reason for the manifestation of individual differences in Figure 16(b). In any case, the phenomenon whereby occurrence of post-apneic snores -when the obstructed airway widens- elicits higher nonstationarity than non-apneic snores during normal breathing, was confirmed for all subjects.

Comparison with Short-time Fourier Transform

Figure 17 shows an example of HHT spectrum (top) and the spectrograms (bo tom) obtained with the Short-time Fourier Transform (STFT) applied to cla 0 snores. In this instance, the analysis window (w) changed to a six-windo format, i.e., 0.0125 seconds, 0.025 seconds, 0.05 seconds, 0.1 seconds, 0.2 se onds, 0.4 seconds, and the time shift was set to 0.0125 seconds. The results fo $w = 0.4$ seconds show the existence of strong peaks around 100 Hz and 300 H However, since the analysis window is too large in this case, the change in th frequency characteristics over time is not identified, and nonstationarity cann be evaluated. Conversely, when $w = 0.0125$ seconds the substantial change i the frequency characteristics over time can be confirmed, and nonstationari can be clearly shown. However, since the resolution of the frequency axis is to coarse, it is not easy to identify the exact frequencies at which the peaks occu

In the HHT spectrum, the time variations of the spectral peaks are not depe dent on this type of trade-off. Accordingly, the peaks for these snoring soun are within the 0.2-0.35 seconds interval, and the frequency can be identified fluctuate in the 100-200 Hz range, which clearly indicates that this is the actu frequency characteristic. Moreover, it also confirms that the frequency fluct ation is considerable around 250-300 Hz. This finding cannot be observed fo any window with width w using STFT, as shown in Figure 17.

In addition, nonstationarity evaluation using average KL is also applied the STFT spectra for comparison. The result is almost the same as that of HH namely, the average KL of class 0 is higher than that of class 1. But HHT is s perior than STFT for analyzing nonstationary properties of post-apneic snore because, when using STFT, it is necessary to adjust the size of the analys window. The window size highly influences nonstationary properties of snor appeared in the spectra, as shown in the bottom of Figure 17. However, de termining the suitable window size, respectively, for each snore episode is daunting task. In the case of HHT, the analysis window itself is theoretical unnecessary, and the instantaneous amplitude of the spectrum can be calculate

Acoustic properties of snores have been considered in relation to speec signals [5–7]. However, Pevernagie et al. [46] state that although speech an snores are similar, they are not equivalent. Therefore, consideration must b given to the difference between them when speech signal processing techniqu are applied. However, they do not outline any specific points of attention. Th

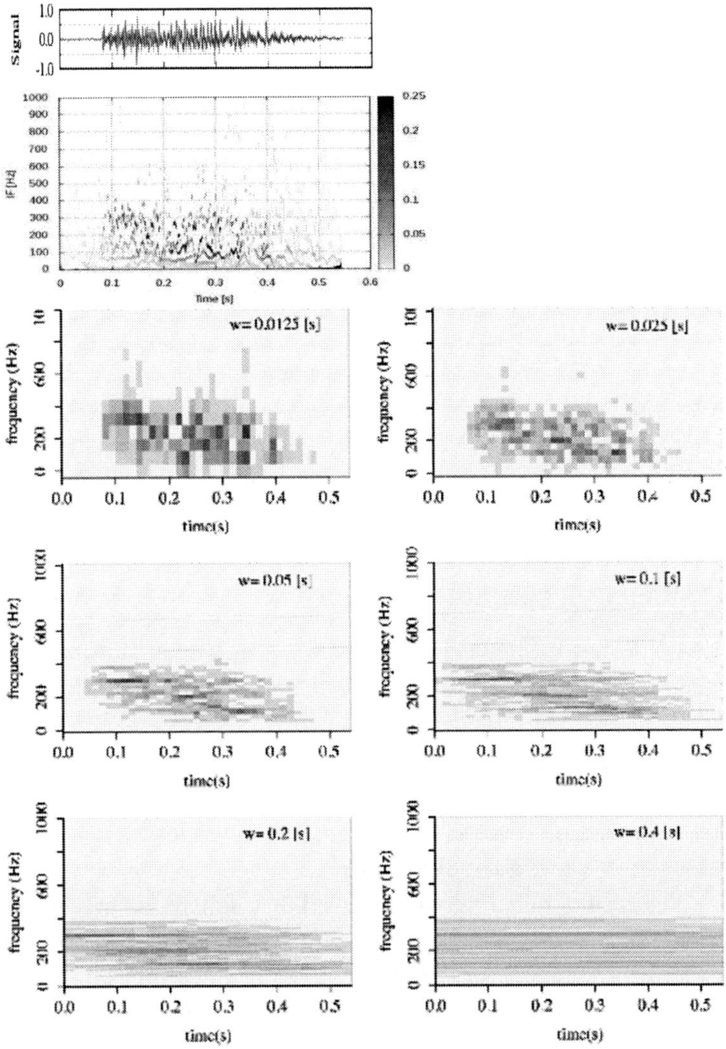

Figure 17. Top: Snoring sound waveform belonging to class 0 and its HHT spectrum. Bottom: Time-frequency spectrograms of class 0 snoring sounds with STFT using various windows for data analyses.

conclusions drawn from the HHT spectra are as follows.

In speech, the sound source is the vibration of the vocal cords, whereas fo snores it is the vibration of the soft palate or the base of the tongue. Sinc the vocal cords are a specific type of hard tissue, stationarity can be assume for their vibration. However, in instances where the sources of vibration ar soft tissues, such as the soft palate, or the base of the tongue, the vibration o the sound source are likely to be affected by the state of the airflow at inspira tion. Correspondingly, it is reasonable to consider that this phase constitutes th phase of primary temporal fluctuation. In the STFT, which is commonly used i speech signal analyses, short-time stationarity is a condition imposed on signa to be analyzed, and vocal cord vibration fulfills this condition. However, fo post-apneic snores which have increased nonstationarity, STFT conditions we not met. The STFT spectrogram in Figure 17 clearly illustrated this finding, an it was virtually impossible to detect the frequency of fluctuation that constitute the cause of the nonstationarity, as indicated in the HHT spectrum in Figure 1

Summary of This Section

A quantitative evaluation was performed to assess the difference between pos apneic snores in OSAS patients that occurred immediately after recovering fro an apnea episode, and non-apneic snores that occurred in non-apneic states i the same patients. The evaluation was conducted based on the degree of no stationarity of acoustic properties. For the quantification, coarse graining wa applied to the plotted HHT spectrograms, followed by the estimation of tempo ral variability using KL divergence.

The results quantitatively showed that nonstationarity was higher for pos apneic snores that occurred immediately after recovery from apnea (class (than for non-apneic snores during normal breathing (class 1) (Figure 16(a) Furthermore, although it was clear that individual differences in these value were substantial, it was revealed that in cases where values were evaluated fo a single subject, a shared characteristic was observed, whereby nonstationari was higher for class 0 than for class 1 (Figure 16(b)). Additional applicatio of this finding promise to contribute to the development of a technique for de tecting severe OSAS from snoring sounds.

Future improvements will include an increase in the number of study sub jects. Additionally, they will incorporate a clarification of the connection wi the morphological characteristics of individual subjects that are related to soft tissues that ultimately increase the severity of OSAS. Moreover, it is possible that decomposed IMFs can represent nonstationary, nonlinear vibrations of multiple vibration sites, and confirmation of states where frequency fluctuates over time. We intend to research the physiological mechanism underlying these processes in more detail in the future.

Conclusion

This chapter focused on the spectral properties of snoring sounds and the morphological properties of oropharyngeal soft tissues in OSAS patients. The authors described some differences among the spectral properties of snoring sounds with three breath routes, and the nonlinear and nonstationary properties of post-apneic snores. As for oropharyngeal soft tissues, the authors evaluated the morphological properties of sagittal tongue and its diagonal elongation is highly related to the severe OSAS. Also, the authors introduced some exception examples of allergic rhinitis, intake of psychoactive medications, and tonsil enlargement. In these cases, it is difficult to recognize OSAS only using sagittal MR images.

Even the PSG, however, cannot avoid the first night effect, leading to a light sleep at sleep laboratory. It is important to detect and diagnose OSAS using other approaches in this case. Then, sound and image-based method in this chapter may become useful for such purpose.

Ethical Approval

Before conducting the analysis described in this chapter, the authors had obtained the permission to use the patients' medical data for the purpose of this study at the Ethical Committee at Hakodate National Hospital.

Acknowledgments

This work was supported in part by JSPS Grant-in-Aid for Scientific Research (C) (Grants No. 26330338 and No. 19K12227; T. Mikami and Grant No.

17K05437; H. Takahashi). This work was also supported in part by Nagaok University of Technology Presidential Research Grant.

REFERENCES

[1] Agnew Jr., H. W., Webb, W. B. & Williams, R. L. (1996). The First Nig Effect: An EEG Study of Sleep. *Psychophysiology*. 2(3), 263-266.

[2] Perez-Padilla, J. R., Slawinski, E., Difrancesco, L. M., Feige, R., Ren mers, J. E. & Whitelaw, W. A. (1993). Characteristics of the Snoring Noi in Patients with and without Occlusive Sleep Apnea. *American Review* *Respiratory Disorders*. 147(3), 635-644.

[3] Fiz, J. A., Abad, J., Jane, R., Riera, M., Mananas, M. A. & Caminal, (1996). Acoustic Analysis of Snoring Sound in Patients with Simple Sno ing and Obstructive Sleep Apnoea. *European Respiratory Journal*. 9(11 2365-2370.

[4] Herzog, M., Schmidt, A., Bremert, T., Herzog, B., Hosemann, W. & Ka tan, H. (2008). Analysed Snoring Sounds Correlate to Obstructive Slee Disordered Breathing. *European Archives of Oto-Rhino-Laryngolog* 265(1), 105-113.

[5] Hara, H., Murakami, N., Miyauchi, Y. & Yamashita, H. (2006). Acoust Analysis of Snoring Sounds by a Multidimensional Voice Program. *Lary goscope*. 116(3), 379-381.

[6] Sola-Soler, J., Jane, R., Fiz, J. A. & Morera, J. (2003). Spectral Env lope Analysis in Snoring Signals from Simple Snorers and Patients wi Obstructive Sleep Apnea. *Proceedings of the 25th Annual Internation Conference of the IEEE Engineering in Medicine and Biology Society*. 2527-2530.

[7] Ng, A. K., Koh, T. S., Baey, E., Lee, T. H., Abeyratne, U. R. & Puv nendran, K. (2008). Could Formant Frequencies of Snore Signals be Alternative Means for the Diagnosis of Obstructive Sleep Apnea? *Slee Medicine*. 9(8), 894-898.

[8] Emoto, T., Abeyratne, U. R., Kusumoto, T., Akutagawa, M., Kondo, E., Kawata, I., Azuma, T., Konaka, S. & Konouchi, Y. (2010). Discriminating Apneic Snorers and Benign Snorers Based on Snoring Formant Extracted via a Noise-robust Linear Prediction Technique. *Journal of Japanese Society for Medical and Biological Engineering*. 48(1), 115-121.

[9] Kitamura, T., Sakabe, A., Ueda, N., Shiomori, T., Udaka, T., Ohbuchi, T. & Suzuki, H. (2008). Usefulness of Cephalometry and Pharyngeal Findings in the Primary Diagnosis of Obstructive Sleep Apnea Syndrome. *Nippon Jibiinkoka Gakkai Kaiho*. 111(11), 695-700.

[10] Yu, X., Fujimoto, K., Urushibata, K., Matsuzawa, Y. & Kubo, K. (2003). Cephalometric Analysis in Obese and Nonobese Patients with Obstructive Sleep Apnea Syndrome. *CHEST*. 124(1), 212-218.

[11] Sakakibara, H., Tong, M., Matsushita, K., Hirata, M., Konishi, Y. & Suetsugu, S. (1999). Cephalometric Abnormalities in Non-obese and Obese Patients with Obstructive Sleep Apnoea. *European Respiratory Journal*. 13(2), 403-410.

[12] Yucel, A., Unlu, M., Haktanir, A., Acar, M. & Fidan, F. (2005). Evaluation of the Upper Airway Cross-sectional Area Changes in Different Degrees of Severity of Obstructive Sleep Apnea Syndrome: Cephalometric and Dynamic CT Study. *American Journal of Neuroradiology*. 26(10), 2624-2629.

[13] Iida-Kondo, C., Yoshino, N., Kurabayashi, T., Mataki, S., Hasegawa, M. & Kurosaki, N. (2006). Comparison of Tongue Volume/Oral Cavity Volume Ratio between Obstructive Sleep Apnea Syndrome Patients and Normal Adults Using Magnetic Resonance Imaging. *Journal of Medical and Dental Science*, 53(2), 119-126.

[14] Schwab, R., Psirstein, M., Pierson, R., Mackley, A., Hachadoorian, R., Areans, R., Maislin, G. & Pack, A. (2003). Identification of Upper Airway Anatomic Risk Factors for Obstructive Sleep Apnea with Volumetric Magnetic Resonance Imaging. *American Journal of Respiratory and Critical Care of Medicine*. 168(5), 522-530.

[15] Arens, R., McDonough, J. M., Corbin, A. M., Hernandez, M. E., Mai lin, G, Schwab, R. I. & Pack, A. I. (2002). Linear Dimensions of tl Upper Airway Structure during Development, Assessment by Magnet Resonance Imaging. *American Journal of Respiratory and Critical Ca Medicine*. 165(1), 117-122.

[16] Mortimore, I. L., Marshall, I., Wraith, P. K., Sellar, R. J. & Douglas, N (1998). Neck and Total Body Fat Deposition in Nonobese and Obese Pa tients with Sleep Apnea Compared with That in Control Subjects. *Amer can Journal of Respiratory and Critical Care Medicine*. 157(1), 280-28

[17] Rodenstein, D., Dooms, G., Thomas, Y., Liistro, G., Stanescu, D. C Culee, C. & Aubert-Tulkens, G. (1990). Pharyngeal Shape and Dimen sions in Healthy Subjects, Snorers, and Patients with Obstructive Slee Apnea. *Thorax*. 45(10), 722-727.

[18] Welch, K. C., Foster, G. D., Ritter, C. T., Wadden, T. A., Arens, R., Mai lin, G. & Schwab, R. J. (2002). A Novel Volumetric Magnetic Resonanc Imaging Paradigm to Study Upper Airway Anatomy. *Sleep*. 25(5), 53 542.

[19] Herrmann, B. L., Wessendorf, T. E., Ajaj, W., Kahlke, S., Teschler, H & Mann, K. (2004). Effects of Octreotide on Sleep Apnoea and Tongu Volume (Magnetic Resonance Imaging) in Patients with Acromegaly. *Eu ropean Journal of Endocrinology*. 151(3), 309-315.

[20] Hoffstein, V. & Mateika, S. (1992). Differences in Abdominal and Nec Circumferences in Patients with and without Obstructive Sleep Apnoe *European Respiratory Journal*. 5(4), 377-381.

[21] Herzog, M., Schieb, E., Bremert, T., Herzog, B., Hosemann, W., Ka tan, H. & Kuhnel, T. (2008). Frequency Analysis of Snoring Sounds du ing Simulated and Nocturnal Snoring. *European Archives of Oto-Rhin Laryngology*. 265 (12), 1553-1562.

[22] Liistro, G., Stanescu, D. & Veriter, C. (1991). Pattern of Simulated Sno ing is Different Through Mouth and Nose. *Journal of Applied Physiolog* 70(6), 2746-2741.

[23] Herzog, M., Metz, T., Schmidt, A., Bremert, T., Venohr, B., Hosemann, W. & Kaftan, H. (2006). The Prognostic Value of Simulated Snoring in Awake Patients With Suspected Sleep-Disordered Breathing: Introduction of a New Technique of Examination. *Sleep*. 29 (11), 1456-1462.

[24] Lofaso, F., Leroux, K., Quera-Salva, M. A., Mroue, G., D'Ortho, M. P., Isabey, D. & Louis, B. (2002). Snoring Detection During Auto-nasal Continuous Positive Airway Pressure. *European Respiratory Journal*. 19(1), 108-112.

[25] Beck, R., Odeh, M., Oliven, A. & Gavriely, N. (1995). The Acoustic Properties of Snores. *European Respiratory Journal*. 8(12), 2120-2128.

[26] Dalmasso, F. & Prota, R. (1996). Snoring: Analysis, Measurement, Clinical Implications and Applications. *European Respiratory Journal*. 9(1), 146-159.

[27] Osborne, J. E., Osman, E. Z., Hill, P. D., Lee, B. V. & Sparkes, C. (1999). A New Acoustic Method of Differentiating Palatal from Non-palatal Snoring. *Clinical Otolaryngology*. 24(2), 130-133.

[28] Heckemann, R. A., Hajnal, J. V., Aljabar, P., Rueckert, D. & Hammers, A. (2006). Automatic Anatomical Brain MRI Segmentation Combining Label Propagation and Decision Fusion. *NeuroImage*. 33(1), 115-126.

[29] Heimann, T., Van Ginneken, B., Styner, M. A., Arzhaeva, Y. et al. (2009). Comparison and Evaluation of Methods for Liver Segmentation from CT Datasets. *IEEE Transactions on Medical Imaging*. 28 (8), 1251-1265.

[30] Hoover, A., Kouznetsova, V. & Goldbaum, M. (2000). Locating Blood Vessels in Retinal Images by Piecewise Threshold Probing of a Matched Filter Response. *IEEE Transactions on Medical Imaging*. 19(3), 203-210.

[31] Lorigo, L. M., Faugeras, O. D., Grimson, W. E. L., Keriven, R., Kikinis, R., Nabavi, A. & Westin, C. F. (2001). CURVES: Curve Evolution for Vessel Segmentation. *Medical Image Analysis*. 5(3), 195-206.

[32] Nakagawa, S. (1999). *Pattern Information Processing*. Maruzen Publisher.

[33] Berry, D. T., Webb, W. B., Block, A. J., Bauer, R. M. & Switzer, D. A (1986). Nocturnal Hypoxia and Neuropsychological Variables. *Journal o Clinical and Experimental Neuropsychology*. 8(3), 229-238.

[34] Young, T., Finn, L. & Kim, H. (1997). Nasal Obstruction as a Risk Facto for Sleep-disordered Breathing. *Journal of Allergy and Clinical Immuno ogy*. 99(2), S757-S762.

[35] Mikami, T., Takahashi, H. & Yonezawa, K. (2019). Detecting Nonlinea and Nonstationary Properties of Post-Apneic Snores using Hilbert-Huan Transform. *Biomedical Engineering: Applications, Basis and Commun cations*. 31(3), 1950017-1-10.

[36] Huang, N. E., Shen, Z., Long, S. R., Wu, M. C., Shih, H. H., Zheng, Q Yen, N. C., Tung C. C. & Liu, H. H. (1998). The Empirical Mode Decom position and the Hilbert Spectrum for Nonlinear and Non-stationary Tim Series Analysis. *Proceedings of the Royal Society A*. 454(1971), 903-99

[37] Salisbury, J. & Sun, Y. (2007). Rapid Screening Test for Sleep Apnea us ing a Nonlinear and Nonstationary Signal Processing Technique. *Medica Engineering & Physics*. 29(3), 336-3443.

[38] Caseiro, P., Fonseca-Pinto, R. & Andrade, A. (2010). Screening of Ob structive Sleep Apnea using Hilbert-Huang Decomposition of Oronasa Airway Pressure Recordings. *Medical Engineering & Physics*. 32(6), 56 568.

[39] Cohen, L. (1995). Time Frequency Analysis: Theory and Application Prentice-Hall, Englewood Cliffs, NJ.

[40] Kaneyama, M., Oohara, K., Takahashi, H., Sekiguchi, Y., Tagoshi, H. & Shibata, M. (2016). Analysis of Gravitational Waves from Binary Neutro Star Merger by Hilbert-Huang Transform. *Physical Review D*. 93, 12301

[41] Wu, Z. & Huang, N. E. (2009). Ensemble Empirical Mode Decompos tion: A Noise-assisted Data Analysis Method. *Advances in Adaptive Da Analysis*. 01(01), 1-49.

[42] Takahashi, H., Oohara, K., Keneyama, M., Hiranuma, Y. & Camp, J. B. (2013). On Investigating EMD Parameters to Search for Gravitational Wave. *Advances in Adaptive Data Analysis*. 05(02), 1350010.

[43] Moreno, P. J., Ho, P. P. & Vasconcelos, N. (2004). A Kullback-leibler Divergence Based Kernel for SVM Classification in Multimedia Applications. *Advances in Neural Information Processing Systems*. 16, 1385.

[44] Ishigaki, T., Higuchi, T. & Watanabe, K. (2007). Deterioration Diagnosis of Pressure Regulator for High Pressure Gas by Spectrum Classification with the Kullback-leibler Kernel. *IEICE Transactions on Information and Systems*. J90(D10), 2789-2797.

[45] Ichioka, M. (2007). Respiratory Organs and Sleep Disorders. *Folia Pharmacolia Japonica*. 129(6), 432-435.

[46] Pevernagie, D., Aarts, R. M. & Meyer, M. D. (2010). The Acoustics of Snoring. *Sleep Medicine Reviews*. 14(2), 131-144.

In: New Research on Sleep …
Editor: Olivier Ratté

ISBN: 978-1-53616-882-2

Chapter 7

APPLICATIONS FOR SMARTPHONE IN SLEEP OBSTRUCTIVE DISORDER BREATHING

A. Battaglia, MD, A. Mistretta, MD, A. Ceraso, MD, S. Gallina*, and F. Lorusso≠, MD

Unit of Otolaringology, Department of Experimental Biomedicine and Clinical Neurosciences, Polyclinic University Hospital "Paolo Giaccone," University of Palermo, Palermo, Italy

ABSTRACT

Today, the technological aspect of the pathology concerning Sleep Obstructive Disorder Breathing, plays an important role. This is due to the growing response in the global population of this issue and given the significant social and financial costs involved in the diagnostic and therapeutic management. Many researchers are moving their attention towards the development of applications for the smartphone related to OSAS, with different purposes: screening app with scientifically accredited issues such as Epworth Sleepness Scale, Stop Bang, Berlin questionnaire; app to monitor the snoring; app to detect the presence of

---

* Professor.
≠ Corresponding Author's E-mail: dott.francescolorusso@gmail.com

apnea; apps with therapeutic purposes. For these kinds of applications, the most important requirements of a smartphone are mainly the presence of a high quality sound card with microphone support and a good accelerometer.

The most downloaded apps on the health theme are those about Sleep Disorders Breathing. These apps can be downloaded with google play or Apple store, some are free but others require payment. This work analyzes and investigates the functionality of the most accredited app available on the actual dowloand for smartphone.

INTRODUCTION

Obstructive breathing disorders in sleep are a common problem in today's society. OSAS is a syndrome that has a significant impact on the quality of life of the person affected, both because of the symptoms it causes and because of possible local and systemic sequelae. One of the problems faced by these disorders is the considerable social and financial costs. In order to carry out a correct diagnosis of OSAS, the use of an adequate instrumental evaluation for the whole night cannot be ignored, but integrated with an appropriate clinical evaluation. In fact, it will be a correct anamnesis aimed at finding symptoms and signs related to an objective specialized examination, to indicate which is the most suitable instrumental method for the selected patient. Hence the importance of adequate phenotype selection to avoid diagnostic errors, excessive costs and waste. A frequent problem encountered by patients is the long waiting lists in public hospitals for polysomnographic monitoring and the excessive costs in the private sector, therefore these two factors often lead people to look for alternative solutions such as the use of specific apps.

Hence the idea throughout the last decade, an undisputed era of smart-phone technology, to try to create applications that could be easy, simple, and cheap to access for patients, for a diagnostic orientation about the alleged disease has been discussed greatly.

The recent increase in the adoption of smartphones by the world community, with increasingly sophisticated sensors, high quality, equipped with advanced systems, has led to the proliferation of many sleep screening applications, developed in collaboration with computer scientists, engineers and doctors. Numerous scientific studies have tried in recent years to understand the possible scientific applicability of such applications. In this chapter we will review the scenario of such applications for smartphones [1].

OPERATION OF THE APPS

You need an operating system to download the apps. The main ones are: Android, RIM, iOS, Windows 7 mobile and Windows Phone 8. The most used are undoubtedly Android and iOS. From the operating system you can dowloand for free or for a fee. Once you have downloaded the application, you can proceed to its use. Applications are based on algorithms and use sensors [2].

- *Microphone-audio system:* A fundamental sensor, present in almost all apps. Audio can be recorded using the smartphone's internal microphone or by placing an external microphone next door. However, the quality of the sound card and microphone provided by your smartphone is important. Once recorded, the audio is processed by the app software to provide metrics or graphs, so as to give the user a qualitative assessment of their sleep. Therefore, it must always be remembered that they do not provide a valid scientific assessment to date. Some apps allow the patient to listen to his snoring recorded throughout the night and to manually identify what would appear to be the most abnormal periods of sleep. Other apps provide an alert noise that alerts the patient when the recorded audio system is above a physiological threshold.
- *Actigraphy and body position:* Actigraphy allows you to reconstruct the pattern of the sleep-wake cycle using an accelerometer. Modern smartphones are equipped with three accelerometers, one for each axis, in order to determine how the

device is moved, and therefore able to provide us with information on body position during sleep. The apps deduct the state of wakefulness or sleep precisely from the body position marked by the accelerometer. In particular, there are some apps that display the incorrect body position, and emit a sound to induce the subject to make an adjustment of the position. They are equipped with an accelerometer that can often be integrated with smartphone apps. It should be remembered, however, that the actigraphy of smartphones is qualitatively different from that of sleep monitoring devices.

- *Video support with camera:* the video function could be used to provide more detailed information on the movement of the subject during the night but currently no app uses this, because there are problems due to the possible need to use infrared for night vision.
- We are studying the *possibility of integrating sensors such as the pulse oximeter.* But this would already make the use of smartphones more investigating and would have higher costs, reducing the accessibility of applications to users.

TYPES OF APP

Among the approximately 100,000,000 health-related apps, there are apps on sleep disorders. By searching, 723 apps were found on Google Play, 593 on the Apple Store. The average price of paid apps was $1.12 at the Apple Store, and $0.58 at Google Play [3].

The contents of these apps can be different:

- apps with screening function;
- snoring monitoring app;
- app to detect the presence of apnea;
- therapeutic apps to reduce snoring and apnea.

In this discussion we will investigate the functionality of the apps most used by users.

Screening Apps

In the literature it is highlighted that the most useful apps regarding apnoea obstructive sleep disorders and snoring are those with scientifically validated screening questionnaires (Epworth scale, Berlin Questionnaire, Stop Bang Questionnaire). These apps are intended to suggest to the patient if exposed to risk of pathology in sleep. From here we can understand how these apps can be for the user the first step that leads to turn to a medical specialist for clinical investigations. One of the most comprehensive apps in this regard is "Screening for Obstructive Sleep Apnea." This app contains the following questionnaires: Epworth Sleepiness Scale Score, Berlin Questionnaire, Stop Bang Questionnaire, Stop Questionnaire Snore Outcome Survery). The user will be able to select the questionnaire, answer the questions and immediately see the score obtained and the consequent stratification of the risk of pathology. The interface is simple and straightforward. It is an app that is useful because the first step of a medical examination is the identification of the risk, which can be evaluated in a first interview just from the answers the patient provides to the doctor through the appropriate questionnaires [3].

The Epworth Sleepiness Scale Score assesses the risk of daytime sleepiness, the user must answer 8 questions relating to daily life, and give each question a score from 0 (zero risk) to 3 (high risk), and finally a score greater than or equal to 11 will put the subject in doubt of being at high risk. The Berlin Questionnaire has three categories of questions, to which the answer must be marked, and if two or more categories were to be positive, poses the risk of being affected by OSAS. Finally, from reviews carried out in the literature, the questionnaire that appears to have the greatest scientific validity is the Stop Bang Questionnaire, designed by Chung et all (2008), for the screening of OSAS risk in patients who are candidates for surgery. This last questionnaire consists of eight questions, to which the user will have to answer with yes or no, and will have to mark his weight and height for the calculation of the BMI, if you answer yes to more than three questions, the user will be at high risk.

APP TO MONITOR SNORING AND APNEA

These are the most popular apps on the market. They monitor the quality of snoring and infer the sleep-wake cycle through the microphone-audio system and the accelerometer. Finally, they report the results in graphic charts, from which it is possible to obtain statistical analyses and make comparisons, analysing the peaks of intensity of the snoring noise detected and seeing the percentage of snoring on the total number of hours of sleep. The position of the smartphone device is important, because the accelerometer used to sense the phase of the sleep cycle of the user is based on the position assumed by the subject during the night.

The higher the quality of the audio-microphone and accelerometer system of the smartphone, the greater the reliability of the results detected [2, 3, 4].

The most downloaded apps on Android and iOS were "Snore Cycle" and "Snore Lab." In "Snore Cycle" you can record the snoring, deduce the sleep cycles from the position assumed on the bed, set the operation of the alarm clocks and finally get a statistical analysis that can be saved on excel file. There is a premium paid function, where you can select annotations, disturbing factors, lifestyle characteristics and monitor your heart rate. "Snore Lab" is an application that has more than a million dowloands especially on Android, and is among the most popular apps. To use it you have to place the app on the bed, set the time of presumed falling asleep and the time of wake-up, and the app will record and monitor the snoring during the night. It will be possible to insert disturbing factors such as caffeine use, smoking, nasal congestion, use of sedatives, dehydration status, pathology and more free of charge, and the app also provides information on possible therapeutic remedies such as oral appliances, c-paps, nasal sprays, nasal dilators, surgery, positional therapy. In the morning you can discover your personal statistics and compare them in the history. Another useful app is "Quit Snoring" which allows you to set the db threshold level and change it, allows you to record sounds and play them back, record the snoring every night and report information on graphs that can be printed and sent by mail, also allows you to mark notes. "Quit Snoring" was the app with the highest score for the sensitivity of the snoring events recording [4].

Other apps with similar features to "Snore Cycle" and "Snore Lab" are "Sleep Time", "Sleepzy", "Sleep as Android", "Smart Alarm Clock", "Sleep Bot", "Sleep Talk Recorder", "Sleep Sounds recorder Plus", "Night Spy", "Dreams Recorder."

Critical issues related to the use of such apps are often the need to place the smartphone in bed, differences in interpretation related to the hardware platform of the device, data loss, delay in data transmission, need to have the device with the battery fully charged and excessive consumption of the use of this, possible hacker attacks and related transmission of personal data, recording of sound sources of other types [5].

Therefore, the user should be properly informed.

Apps for Therapeutic Purposes

There are apps that attempt to provide therapeutic support by activating a light and/or sound and/or vibratory signal as soon as the device signals snoring. The app "Anti snoring lite" sends either a loud sound signal or a bright flash or a strong vibration as soon as the snoring is detected, in the paid version allows you to select all three types of anti-snoring alarm. The problem with this app is that it does not distinguish snoring from coughing or disturbing voices, as it will be activated by any sound that exceeds the db threshold, and it is advisable to place the phone near the head. There are apps that try to help you fall asleep by sending relaxing sounds that help you sleep. The app "Relax Melodies" allows you to select the type of sound most favorable for falling asleep, such as the chirping of birds, the sound of rain or wind, a pleasant melody.

CONCLUSION

Studies in the literature have tried to evaluate the scientific validity and clinical applicability of smartphone apps but to date has not been found scientific validity, there are no clear answers, further studies are needed to understand this. It is important, however, to reiterate the concept that a smart-phone device cannot and must not replace the doctor. Technology can be a great help for the scientific community and for patients, in fact such apps can help a user to understand if he is at risk of OSAS disease, can provide information on the disease and any therapeutic possibilities, can help to understand how to change life habits by eliminating disturbing factors, can allow you to become aware of a problem by listening to audio recordings of your snoring, and allows you to have personal statistics to compare, but what is important is that you know how to use them with proper orientation and correct criteria, without ever ergerarle to replace appropriate specialist examination.

REFERENCES

[1] Grigsby-Toussaint DS, Shin JC, Reeves DM, Beattie A, Auguste E, Jean-Louis G. Sleep apps and behavioral constructs: A content analysis. *Prev. Med. Rep.* 2017 Feb 21;6:126-129.

[2] Behar J, Roebuck A, Domingos JS, Gederi E, Clifford GD. A review of current sleep screening applications for smartphones. *Physiol. Meas.* 2013 Jul;34(7):R29-46.

[3] Ong AA, Gillespie MB. Overview of smartphone applications for sleep analysis. *World J. Otorhinolaryngol Head Neck Surg.* 2016 Mar 5;2(1):45-49.

[4] Camacho M, Robertson M, Abdullatif J, Certal V, Kram YA, Ruoff CM, Brietzke SE, Capasso R. Smartphone apps for snoring. *J. Laryngol. Otol.* 2015 Oct;129(10):974-9.

[5] Ong AA, Gillespie MB. Overview of smartphone applications for sleep analysis. *World J. Otorhinolaryngol. Head Neck Surg.* 2016 Mar 5;2(1):45-49.

In: New Research on Sleep …
Editor: Olivier Ratté
ISBN: 978-1-53616-882-2

Chapter 8

THE ROLE OF SURGERY IN THE TREATMENT OF OSAS

***F. Lorusso**, *MD, A. Battaglia, MD, A. Mistretta, MD and S. Gallina*≠**

Unit of Otolaringology, Department of Experimental Biomedicine and Clinical Neurosciences, Polyclinic University Hospital "Paolo Giaccone", University of Palermo, Palermo, Italy

ABSTRACT

The American Academy of Sleep Medicine [1] and the American Academy of Otolaryngology–Head and Neck Surgery [2] recommend surgery as an option for the treatment of OSAS, when non-invasive treatments such as CPAP or oral appliances have not been successful or are not tolerated. Surgical treatment is more effective when there is an evident anatomical deformity that can be corrected to alleviate the respiratory obstruction.

According to the American Sleep Apnea Association, a gradual and logical approach must be taken into account when a patient seeks a

---

* Corresponding Author's E-mail: dott.francescolorusso@gmail.com.
≠ Professor.

surgical solution, and it is a fundamental requirement that the patient find a surgeon who understands both the pathophysiology of sleep apnea and anatomy of the upper airways (UA) to guarantee the best chances of success [3].

The surgical options aim to solve the obstructive problem according to two ways, the first is the reduction of the content, and then acts through the volumetric reduction of soft tissues at the level of UA, most often at the level of palate, uvula, tonsils, adenoids and tongue. The second option aims at enlarging the container, and therefore on more complex interventions to adapt the bony structures of the skull.

Surgical interventions can be schematically divided into nasal surgery, oropharyngeal surgery, hypopharyngeal surgery, laryngeal surgery, multilevel surgery and upper airway by-pass.

The soft palate in the snore-surgery is the anatomical site on which most of the attention has always been concentrated since it is responsible for most of the phenomena of snoring and most of the obstructive ones and has undergone the greatest innovations.

The rationale for palatal surgery is to reduce volume and stiffen a structure that vibrating with the passage of air causes snoring and collapsing causes an obstruction of the UA.

In general, interventions on the palate can be broadly divided into two groups, the first is represented by interventions that have the aim of reduce snoring, and in this case are less invasive surgeries, as the goal is that of stiffening the palate and reducing the excess mucosa that vibrating causes snoring.

The second group consists of interventions that have the aim of reducing above the snoring especially the apnoic episodes, so they are interventions that have a greater invasiveness, since they must stiffen and reconstitute the functionality of a segment of the UA.

In this context, in the last few years great importance has been placed in the surgeon of the oropharynx side wall starting from the Cahali techniques [4], followed by the Exphansion Sphincter Pharingoplasty by Pang and Woodson [5] up to the innovative techniques such as the Barbed Reposition Pharingoplasty of Vicini and Mantovani [6].

Surgical Treatment

The American Academy of Sleep Medicine [1] and the American Academy of Otolaryngology–Head and Neck Surgery [2] recommend surgery as an option for the treatment of OSAS, when non-invasive treatments such as CPAP or oral appliances have not been successful or are not tolerated. Surgical treatment is more effective when there is an evident anatomical deformity that can be corrected to alleviate the respiratory obstruction.

According to the American Sleep Apnea Association, a gradual and logical approach must be taken into account when a patient seeks a surgical solution, and it is a fundamental requirement that the patient find a surgeon who understands both the pathophysiology of sleep apnea and anatomy of the upper airways (UA) to guarantee the best chances of success [3].

The surgical options aim to solve the obstructive problem according to two ways, the first is the reduction of the content, and then acts through the volumetric reduction of soft tissues at the level of UA, most often at the level of palate, uvula, tonsils, adenoids and tongue. The second option aims at enlarging the container, and therefore on more complex interventions to adapt the bony structures of the skull.

Fundamental assumptions are:

- the patient must be highly motivated and must express the desire to carry out the treatment,
- treatment should not damage the patient and after any treatment nasal ventilatory therapy should remain possible,
- surgical treatment must be planned according to the patient's specific anatomical characteristics and the severity of the syndrome.
- As with all other treatment modalities, there is no surgical intervention that can guarantee a certainty of a stable result over time.
- More serious is the OHSAS, more complex and challenging it is the effective intervention.
- In any case we will try to opt for the minimum effective solution able to manage the severity of the complained disorder.

Nasal surgery:

- Septoplasty
- Functional rhinoplasty, nasal valve surgery

- Turbinate surgery
- Adenoidectomy
- Nasal polypectomy
- Endoscopic procedure

Oropharyngeal surgery:

- Tonsillectomy
- Palatal surgery (uvulectomy and pharyngoplasty)
- Minimally invasive surgery (RF, pillar, sclerotherapy)

Hypopharyngeal surgery:

- Hyoid suspension
- Lingual surgery (tongue reductions, glossectomies and TORS)
- Advancement of genioglossus
- Mandibular advancement

Laryngeal surgery:

- Epiglottectomy
- Supraglottoplasty

UA by-pass:

- Tracheostomy

Global procedures:

- Bi-maxillary advancement
- Multilevel surgery
- Bariatric surgery

Nasal Surgery

The relationship between sleep disorder breathing (SDB) and nasal function is complex, in fact the nose is not only an obstructive site, but it also has considerable influence on the most downstream sites because a difficult nasal breathing creates an increase in negative pressure at the level of the pharyngeal tract it is more collapsible. If the obstruction is such that it does not allow an adequate air flow, it causes the necessary passage to oral breathing, with consequent worsening of the obstruction linked to the lingual and hypopharyngeal component.

There are many interventions aimed at improving nasal breathing, but none of these is considered alone as osas surgery, as the improvement of nasal breathing can also drastically reduce the signs and symptoms associated with SDB, but in most cases the benefit is partial.

- Septoplasty
- Decongestion of inferior turbinates
- Turbinoplasty
- Polypectomy or endoscopic surgery
- Functional rhinoplasty, nasal valve surgery

The results on snoring are often controversial and are also difficult to interpret because often there is an improvement of the noise, since they reduce the constrictions and the vortical flows at the nasal level responsible for the nasal snoring. But in other cases there may be a worsening of the symptomatology due to the greater vibration of the soft tissues of the most downstream sites linked to the greater air flow established thanks to the surgery.

Usually the improvement of nasal breathing is associated with an improvement in the quality of sleep and daytime vigilance. The results on the OSAS are however partial and aleatory.

Only Rubin and coll. [7] in their study achieved a significant improvement in OSAS severity only with nasal surgery, while remaining far from the parameters of surgical success. In subjects with mild OSAS, nasal tamponade is usually not a problem. But in patients with moderate to severe OSAS, nasal tamponade can precipitate respiratory failure in post-surgery. Therefore, in these cases it would be appropriate to use medications that allow nasal breathing through appropriate channels. The most risky period is represented by the first 6 hours post-surgery [7], therefore in this period the patient should be constantly monitored. In subjects with severe OSAS who have already undergone CPAP therapy and who must necessarily receive post-operative nasal tamponade, it is recommended to resume post-operative CPAP therapy immediately, either with a facial mask or an oral mask.

The importance of nasal surgery in improving nCPAP compliance should not be forgotten [8].

Friedman et al. [9] in a group of patients undergoing septoplasty and lower turbinoplasty reported a reduction in CPAP pressure required to resolve OSAS from 9.3 mbar to 6.7 mbar. Dorn and coll. [10] showed a reduction in CPAP of 3.2 mbar, 6 weeks after nasal surgery.

Rhinopharyngeal Surgery

If an obstacle is detected, its ablation is indicated here, but assumptions and expectations are similar to those of nasal surgery. The most frequent causes are adenoid hypertrophy and rarely antrocoanal polyps in children, while in adults there are rarely obstructions at this level. Should this occur, attention must be paid to the risks of scarring stenosis in case of a contemporary adenoidectomy to palatal surgery, in fact it is not recommended by many authors to make it in a single time.

In children, adenoid hypertrophy contributes to the determinism of childhood SDB. But adenoidectomy is not sufficient to solve the OSAS problem, but together with tonsillectomy it is considered the primary therapy for the resolution of infant SDB. [11] Adenoidectomy is to be considered only in simple snoring in fact it is known in children a strong relationship between the adenoid dimension and snoring [12, 13]. Nieminen et al. [14] in a prospective non-randomized controlled trial evaluated with PSG a group of children subjected to adenoidectomy before and after surgery, 73% of these did not resolve the obstructive problem or symptoms started after adenoidectomy, probably due to compensatory tonsil hypertrophy.

Oropharyngeal Surgery

The oropharynx is the anatomical site with the most important role in the ronco-surgery as it is located at the carrefour between the oral and nasal respiratory tract, and it is mostly at this level that due to the considerable presence of loose structures there is the greatest influence on the obstruction of the UA.

Therefore, the objectives of the ronco-surgery at this level are two [15]:

1. Reduction/abolition of vibrating tissue responsible for snoring;
2. Reduction/abolition of the obstructing tissue responsible for RERAs, hypopneas and apnea.

Tonsil Surgery

Child's Tonsillar Ronco-Surgery

Tonsillar hypertrophy is the main cause of OSAS and snoring in the pediatric population [16-18]. The age of less than three years, neurological and maxillofacial comorbidity are to be assessed with care and caution for an increased post-operative risk and for a greater share of failures. The opportunity for post-operative monitoring in pediatric intensive care units should be considered in this group of patients.

Various techniques have been developed that can be basically divided into two basic types of intervention:

- *Tonsillotomy or tonsillar volumetric reduction:* which consists in reducing the volume of the tonsils, with preservation of their capsule, which can be performed with various instruments such as coblator, microdebrider, radiofrequency. This technique appears to be burdened with a lower risk of post-operative bleeding [19]. But it presents the risk of recurrence of hypertrophy.

- *Tonsillectomy*: which consists in the complete removal of the tonsil with its capsule, it can be performed with cold techniques or with hot techniques [20]. These latter techniques are burdened from a slightly higher risk of post-operative late hemorrhage 2-4%, compared to 1-2% of cold techniques [21].

The almost total disappearance of night snoring after adeno-tonsillectomy in children is widely known, but there are only a few studies to prove it.

The work of Hultcranz et al. Is interesting in this regard [22] that in a randomized study compared the effectiveness on tonsillectomy and tonsillotomy snoring after one year, showing a 9.5% recurrence of snoring in the group of patients undergoing tonsillotomy, suggesting a possible relapse hypertrophy.

Adenotonsillectomy is considered the first line treatment in the treatment of pediatric OSAS [2, 15, 24-27].

Brietzke [28] in his meta-analysis has shown how obesity is a fundamental factor in the determinism of the presence of post-surgical OSAS residue. Finding an AHI> 5 sleep events/hour in 59% of obese children subjected to adenotonsillectomy. And highlighting as predisposing factors in the maintenance of a post-operative high AHI age> 7 aa, the presence of asthma and a severe preoperative OSAS, in all these cases the child must undergo post-operative polysomnography, to evaluate the possible presence of residual OSAS.

In an attempt to reduce post-operative pain, various devices have been developed, which in most cases aim to achieve the simplicity of a tonsillectomy with hot instruments while maintaining contained temperatures of use. From this point of view we conducted a comparative study between tonsillectomy for cold dissection and tonsillectomy with Molecular Quantum Resonance, results showed a saving in surgical time and a significant reduction in intra-operative bleeding, although not having significant results with regard to post-operative pain that was substantially overlapping [20].

Adult's Tonsillar Surgery

The hypertrophic palatine tonsil is a significant obstacle at the VAS level, easily eliminated with relatively rudimentary surgery, but usually this is not sufficient to completely solve the snoring and OSAS problem. As evidenced by Tzifa and coll. [29] tonsillectomy in children does not reduce the risk of becoming snoring adults. Rarely in the surgical treatment of snoring and OSAS is it limited only to tonsillectomy, but when this procedure is performed within a multisite procedure the contribution of tonsillar time to overall success appears to be relevant. This is also due to the fact that an important tonsillar hypertrophy is rare in the adult subject, but when this happens the tonsillectomy has a success rate similar to that of the pediatric age.

Tonsillar Volumetric Reduction Radio-Frequencies

The principle consists in the submucosal application of low frequency radio waves. It is used as an interstitial treatment, with an electrode that is inserted into the soft tissue of the tonsil creating a thermal lesion that causes necrosis and is followed by successive cicarizial processes. As a consequence, the soft tissue shrinks and stiffens. [19, 30].

Palatal Surgery

The soft palate in otolaryngology surgery is the anatomical site on which most of the attention has always been concentrated since it is responsible for most of the snoring phenomena and a good part of the obstructive ones.

The rationale of palatal surgery is to reduce volume and stiffen a structure that vibrates with the passage of air causing snoring and collapsing causes an obstruction of the UA.

Generally, interventions on the palate can be broadly divided into two groups, the first is represented by treatments that aim to reduce snoring, and in this case they are less invasive surgical interventions, as the goal is that of stiffening the palate and reducing the excess mucosa that vibrates, causeing snoring. The second group is made up of the treatments that aim to reduce the apnoic episodes above snoring, therefore they are surgical interventions that have a greater invasiveness, since they must stiffen and rebuild the functionality of a segment of the UA.

- Treatment of Snoring

Uvulectomy

In literature there are few results regarding the uvulectomy as a single surgical treatment for the treatment of snoring. It is a very painful procedure and is not recommended, except for removing the exuberant mucosa, especially if you are going to resect the muscular component of the uvula. As demonstrated by Mortimore [31], mere resection of the uvula increases oral bleeding in patients undergoing CPAP.

Radiofrequency (RF) Snoreplasty

In 1995 Whinney et al. suggested a procedure considered to be a precursor to soft palatal RF, using diathermocoagulation of the palatal muscles by infixion [23]. The use of RF has made it possible to considerably reduce thermal damage. The procedure is usually performed under local anesthesia with the patient in a sitting position. But it can also be associated with other nasal procedures or tonsillectomy and is therefore performed in the context of a general anesthesia.

There are numerous studies on the effectiveness of RF on snoring with an average improvement of about 82.4%. The most frequent complications are burn, erosion and ulceration of the lining mucosa. This phenomenon, however, besides causing a greater post-operative pain, usually does not affect the final result since, if the lesion is only on the ventral side of the palate, it creates a greater scarring reaction that makes the palate more rigid. On the other hand, excessively deep thermal lesions that cause damage to the mucous membrane of the dorsal side of the palate are to be avoided, causing an alteration of the healing dynamics.

Certainly effective on simple snoring, it can also be effective in mild OSAS, both as a single technique on the palate and in a minimally invasive multilevel surgery.

Injection Snoreplasty

The rational is similar to that of the RF, only that instead of the thermal stimulus, sclerosing substances are used to induce the formation of scars on the palate. Introduced for the first time in 2001 by Brietzke [33], initially using a 3% solution of sodium tetradecyl sulfate (STS). Provided after local anesthesia at sub-mucosal level, and within a few weeks the mucosa undergoes healing. Transient improvement in snoring has been reported.

Palatal Implants

They consist of small polyethylene splints (PET) similar to that used for vascular endoprostheses or gastric meshes. Three of these are applied under local anesthesia thanks to a special applicator in the context of the palatal musculature, stimulating a fibrotic reaction that creates a capsule around the implant with the aim of stiffening the palate reducing its vibration.

The technique has been virtually abandoned in the light of poor clinical results encountered and of the rare, but still detected episodes of implant expulsion with a percentage from 0 to 25% [34].

Velo-Uvulo-Pharyngeal Lift (VUPL)

In 2008 Hur [35] proposed a technique of snoreplasty based on the stiffening of the redundant soft tissues of the soft palate through the trans-mucosa introduction of permanent sutures through the fibro-muscular plane of the palate. This study achieved poor results on the OSAS, but highlighted the perfect tolerability of these sutures, already widely used in plastic surgery, at the palatal level, allowing to obtain the desired modifications in the fibro-muscular tissues surrounded by the sutures. In 2012 Mantovani and coll. [36], have developed a new palatal lifting technique using non-resorbable sutures, the so-called "Roman blinds" technique. This has the aim not only to make the veil-uvular complex rise and stiffen, but also making it advance also widens the mesopharyngeal space to eliminate the noisy vibrations or occlusions. The technique involves the use of non-absorbable 2-0 sutures that are anchored with different passages to three bony structures (the two pterygoid hamuli, and the posterior nasal spine), through a small mucosal incision and then in a loop inside the palatopharyngeal fibro-muscular tissues. The side effects of the technique were limited to post-operative pain that disappears rapidly within a few days. Subsequently the technique has been further implemented [37] with the use of barbed wires (QUill ® Knotless Tissue Closure Device, Angiotech Pharmaceutical inc., Vancouver, CA), normally used in vascular surgery, which do not require knots, as they are self-locking and allow you to get new geometries.

- Treatment of Apnea

The first plastic coded intervention of the soft palate was described for the first time by Ikematsu in 1963, since then numerous interventions have been proposed that aim to reduce the excess components of the soft palate tissue, without compromising the swallowing and phonatory functions. In fact the palatoglossus muscle (anterior palatal pillar) contains within it neuro-muscular spindles, playing an important role in swallowing and therefore must be preserved together with the muscle of the uvula.

While the glossopharyngeal muscle (posterior palatal pillar) has no neuro-muscular spindles, therefore, it can be partially dissected without hindering swallowing or the possibility of a future nasal ventilatory therapy (nCPAP). In fact, an excessive resection of the palatal musculature creates serious difficulties in the application of nCPAP due to oral venting. A fundamental prerequisite of palatal surgery is the implementation of techniques that make it possible to maintain CPAP in any case as a therapeutic alternative in the event of failure.

Indications and contraindications are similar for all palatal interventions to reduce apnea.

Indications for exclusive palatal intervention:

- Hypertrophic and elongated uvula (dolico-mega-uvula)
- Palatine Ptosis
- Thick palate
- Tonsillar hypertrophy

- Restricted oropharyngeal isthmus
- Plication of the pharyngeal walls
- BMI <30
- AHI <20 or simple snoring

Absolute contraindications of palatal surgery:

- Cleft palate
- Short palate
- Insufficient oral opening, interdental distance <3 cm (small operating field)
- Chronic cardiac or pulmonary disorders
- Neurological or psychiatric disorders requiring pharmacological treatment
- High anesthetic risk
- Alcoholism
- Sedative abuse
- Skull facial anomalies

Contraindications to treatment with palatal surgery only:

- Obesity: generally represents a negative selection criterion. But only palatal intervention with BMI> 30 is contraindicated
- severe OSAS, AHI> 30 also 20 according to some authors
- Retrognathia or micrognathia (usually lingual back obstruction)
- Severe occlusal or temporomandibular joint dysfunction (oral opening <3cm)
- High distance between the hyoid and lower edge of the jaw

Relative contraindications of palatal surgery:

- Professional use of the voice
- Wind instrument players

- Scuba diving activities (possible problems of tubal compensation)
- Professional use of taste

Uvulo Palato Pharyngoplasty (UPP or UP3)

The original technique was first described by Ikematsu in 1963, since then numerous variants have been proposed, as long as UPPP is to be considered as a group of procedures.

The first UPPs included a very aggressive resection of the soft palate with frequent complications such as velo-farinea insufficiency 24% [38], 4% nasopharyngeal stenosis [39] and frequent failure to use nCPAP due to oral venting [40]. Therefore these techniques have been globally abandoned.

UPP is effective in the resolution of snoring of velar origin.

Hassid et al. [41] have recently described a decrease in success rates with increasing follow-up periods.

A polysomnographic follow-up is recommended after 1-3 aa. From the data it is clear that the effectiveness of UPPP decreases over the years. Using the Sher success criteria as a parameter (AHI reduction> 50% and values <20) [42], a long-term success rate of 49.5% is achieved.

According to the AASM in patients with moderate-severe OSAS, UPPP with or without tonsillectomy does not allow a normalization of the AHI therefore should be proposed only after a manifest refusal of treatment with CPAP or oral appliances [43].

The effectiveness of the surgery is not proportional to the size of the resection while the side effects and risks are directly proportional to the size of the resection [15].

Mortimore [31] has shown that an aggressive resection of the velar muscles during UPPP does not allow the application of nCPAP at pressures greater than 13 cm of H2O.

Excessive aggression on the side walls and post-operative infections are the main cause of nasopharyngeal strictures.

Uvulo-Palatal Flaps

Palatal flaps are generally an interesting alternative to UPPP and are indicated for primary snoring and mild to moderate OSAS. Post-operative pain is less than UP3. The operation is always preceded by tonsillectomy, in the case of tonsillectomized patients unlike UPPP the scar tissue should not be removed to highlight the pharyngeal palate muscle that should not be dissected here. The tip of the uvula must be pulled down and an incision is made about 2 cm away from the contact point represented by the junction between the hard palate and the soft palate. At this point part of the redundant mucosa is removed at the level of the anterior aspect of the soft palate together with the distal part of the muscle of the uvula, making a posterior mucous flap which, depending on the techniques, may have a rectangular or triangular shape.

This is in turn tipped forward and sutured to the edges of the incision. Depending on the techniques, more or less abundant resections of the uvula or incisions of the soft palate can also be performed. Then the two palatine pillars are sutured together if tonsillectomy was performed. This flap must have an adequate thickness in so as to avoid that the new palate is excessively thick. A possible dehiscence of the sutures creates functional and subjective difficulties. The duplication of the flap on a palate is often not without functional and subjective problems.

There are few data in the literature regarding the treatment of snoring, while there is some study about the treatment of OSAS, but from the limited data available and the extreme similarity of the technique to the more conservative UPPP is possible to assume that they have comparable results.

Laser Uvulopalatoplasty (LUPP) and Laser Assisted Uvulopalatoplasty (LAUP)

The LUPP introduced by Carenfelt [44] in the late 1980s was similar to classical UPPP under general anesthesia, but used the CO2 laser for incisions. In 1990 Kamami [45] completely modified the technique, developing a procedure under local anesthesia in several sessions called LAUP. This technique in the 90s due to its simplicity of application has quickly taken off in Europe and the USA, with the appearance of innumerable variants. In general, the technique involves two paramedian incisions of the palate, at full thickness, from both sides of the uvula with a height of 1-2 cm. And a total or partial uvulectomy. The technical variants include variants in which the intervention was performed in a single step and variants performed in different sessions. Subsequently some authors, given the scarce results obtained and the frequent complications, started to develop more conservative techniques on the palatal musculature, removing only the mucosa at the palatoglossus muscle level, while the uvula and the posterior pillar were treated as in the LUPP or LAUP [46]. From the results obtained, the LAUP was less effective than UPPP in the reduction of snoring, nocturnal awakenings, daytime sleepiness and apneas. It is also a very painful technique and in multi-step procedures about 20% of patients refused to undergo another session because of pain [22]. Furthermore the complications were very frequent.

Therefore, due to poor results and frequent side effects from the early 2000s, LUPP and LAUP are not recommended as surgical procedures. In 2001, the Standards of Practice Committee of the American Academy of Sleep Medicine issued some guidelines regarding the LAUP advising against its use [23].

Lateral Pharingoplasty (LP)

It is the first technique to pay significant attention to the role of the lateral wall of the pharynx in the determinism of the OSAS. Developed by Cahali [32] in 2003 it has as a fundamental premise the stiffening of the lateral wall of the pharynx. In fact the obstruction linked to the lateral walls of the pharynx is the only risk factor, besides BMI and neck circumference, which acts independently in the determinism of the OSAS in man [48].

Cahali in the indications inserted the presence of at least two of the following characteristics:

- Lateral peritonsillar narrowing (defined as the size of peritonsillar tissues greater than 25% of the pharyngeal space, calculated as the internal distance of the mandible measured in the middle of the tonsillar fossa);

- tonsillar hypertrophy (defined as lateral bulkiness of the tonsils greater than 50% of the distance between the posterior tonsillar pillars);
- ptosic soft palate (which does not allow visualization of the posterior pharyngeal wall).

In addition to these assumptions, the subjects had to present to the fiber optic pharyngoscopy a narrowing or collapse in the retropalatal region without narrowing in the hypopharynx, both at rest and during the Müller maneuver.

The first step of the surgical procedure is tonsillectomy with identification of the palatoglossus and palatofaingeo muscle. Then they identify and raise the fibers of the upper constrictor muscle of the pharynx at the level of the tonsillar fossa, as far as possible from the glossopharyngeal. Once detached from the lateropharyngeal space, the upper pharynx constrictor is sectioned in a cranio-caudal direction obtaining two muscular flaps. The medial flap is left in situ, while the lateral flap is sutured anterior to the palatoglossus muscle. Then a Z-plastic is made between the mucosa of the anterior aspect of the soft palate and the upper portion of the palate-pharyngeal muscle, covering the upper part of the tonsillar fossa, while the lower part of the loggia is closed by suturing the remaining part of the pharyngeal palate muscle to the anterior pillar.

With the suspension to the palatoglossus muscle Cahali tries to give support to the oropharynx and the tongue. While with the Z plastic, he tries to orient the scar retraction laterally.

The technique has several side effects such as persistent pain, reflux of fluids from the nose. But the main complication due to the section of the upper pharyngeal constrictor is lasting dysphagia especially for solids.

In a subsequent article Cahali [48] reports the improvement of post-operative swallowing recovery with the preservation of the stylopharyngeal muscle that was frequently sacrificed. But the main risk is related to the section of the upper pharynx constrictor is the exposure of the parapharyngeal space with its important neuro-vascular structures.

Expansion Sphincter Pharyngoplasty (ESP)

Even ESP is based on the fundamental concept that at pharyngeal level the obstruction linked to the collapse of the lateral walls of the pharynx plays a fundamental role. This technique was developed by Pang and Woodson in 2007 [49], and is currently one of the most applied pharyngoplasty, even by our group [50], since it is effective and less invasive than lateral pharyngoplasty.

The main indications are:

- Predominantly lateral pharyngeal collapse
- Wide and thick posterior pillars
- Thick soft palate

It has specific contraindications, in addition to the general ones for palatal surgery, in the event of:

- Absence of lateral pharyngeal collapse
- Tonsillary pillars fused together
- Very thin soft palate
- Scar palate

The first step of the surgery consists in bilateral tonsillectomy with identification of the palato-glosso and palato-pharyngeal muscle and preservation of the covering mucosa. The palato-pharyngeal muscle is then isolated from the surrounding tissues, preserving the fibers of the upper pharyngeal constrictor. At this point, two ligatures are placed at the level of the distal margin of the muscle, to keep the muscle fibers together and to ensure better hemostasis, since the muscle is sectioned downwards creating a superior hinged muscle flap, in part connected to the upper constrictor of the pharynx.

At this point, the original technique involves an incision of the palato-glossus muscle fibers at the palatine arch plane and the suture of the distal portion of the flap at this level, and the subsequent suturing of the superficial mucous planes. In our experience this passage was modified by creating a tunnel with a klemmer forceps in the context of the soft palate with a 45° angle in the direction of the pterigoid hamulus, tipping the muscular flap inside the tunnel and fixing it with two resorbable stitches in position, obtaining an antero-lateral palate stretching [50]. At this point the palatine pillars are joined with a resorbable suture. A partial uvulectomy is performed depending on the laxity of the uvular mucosa.

Patients are monitored post-operatively for a few hours with pulso-oximetry and an adequate pain therapy is administered, since for the first post-operative week there is pain on swallowing.

Pang et al. do not report complications such as reflux of fluids from the nose or palatal insufficiency, palatal fistulas or oral infections. Which did not even occur in our experience. But unlike the author we reported 2 cases of post-operative haemorrhage, occurring in the first operations, probably linked to the inevitable learning curve.

The key points of the surgery are:

- The increased space at the transverse level at the level of the pharynx both for the removal of the tonsils and for the dislocation of the palato-pharyngeal muscle
- The incomplete isolation of the palato-pharyngeal muscle from the upper pharyngeal constrictor thanks to which it creates sufficient tension on the side walls
- ESP also tends to widen further, in the anterolateral sense, the space at the level of the oropharyngeal vestibule during the healing phases, since the cicatricial retraction of the palate-pharyngeal muscle flap stretches the palate and the lateral walls of the pharynx even more in this sense by creating centrifugal healing vectors. Contrary to UPPP where the healing vectors were centripetal with a progressive worsening of the results obtained.

Pang et al. [49] showed a significant improvement in AHI compared to UPPP, with a percentage of surgical success according to the Sher criteria of 82.6% for ESP against 68.1% for UPPP, with a significant difference in oropharyngeal transverse diameters post-operative where after ESP the residual transverse collapse with Muller maneuver was modest, while after UPPP it was still very evident.

In our experience ESP has proved to be an effective weapon in the management of palatal obstruction. In fact in patients subjected exclusively to ESP due to the presence of a predominantly palatal obstructive site, an improvement in AHI was obtained, which on average was reduced by 63.4% with a success rate according to the Sher criteria of 65% [50]. We have also shown in all patients subjected to ESP a notable improvement as regards the anatomical parameters at the oropharyngeal level. In fact, a notable dilatation of the transverse diameters and a progression of the palate considerably higher than the UPPP, with a reduction of the oropharyngeal collapse to the Müller maneuver equal to 64.7%.

Relocation Pharyngoplasty

This technique introduced in 2009 by Li and coll. [51], based on the increase in the volume of the pharyngeal vestibule acting on the lateral walls of the pharynx, with a technique similar to that of Cahali [32]. After tonsillectomy with careful conservation of the mucosa of the palatine pillars. The pharyngeal palate muscle is taken near the uvula and rotated upwards and sideways making it approach the remaining part of the soft palate.

The full-thickness tissue of two elliptical zones at the level of the soft palate is removed, including mucosa, submucosa, adipose tissue and muscle. The upper pharyngeal constrictor is sutured to the homolateral palatoglossus muscle with a cranio-caudal direction. The palatal-pharyngeal muscle is separated from the upper constrictor of the pharynx to facilitate tension-free approximation. The pharyngeal palate muscle with its mucous flap is then anteriorized and also sutured on the palatoglossus muscle. Finally, a partial uvulectomy is planned.

With this technique a single, rigid and anterior newly formed palatine is created, which puts the lateral walls of the pharynx in tension and increases the posterior space because the advancement of the posterior pillar also brings with it the dorsal portion of the palate.

The results show a significant reduction in snoring of daytime sleepiness and AHI. No post-operative bleeding, reflux of liquids from the nose or alterations of the voice were found.

This technique, unlike that of Cahali, does not involve a dissection of the upper pharyngeal constrictor with consequent opening of the lateropharyngeal space and the risk of damaging the important neuro-vascular structures contained in it.

Anterior Pharyngoplasty

It consists of a technique of palatal tightening introduced for the first time by Pang in 2008 [52], indicated in the treatment of snoring and mild-moderate OSAS associated with tonsillectomy. Pang performed the procedure under local anesthesia if it was not associated with tonsillectomy in the case of absent or small tonsils (grade 0-2) or in general anesthesia when associated with tonsillectomy (grade 3-4 tonsils). In our experience we have always preferred to carry out surgery under general anesthesia.

The technique consists in practicing a partial uvulectomy, removing only the mucosa. Followed by the removal of a rectangle of anterior mucosa of the palate about 40-50 mm long and 7-10 mm high, until the underlying musculature is uncovered. And then after haemostasis, the two upper and lower flaps are gathered together with absorbable sutures anchored at full thickness in the musculature of the palate, creating an elevation and anteriorization of the palate. Pang reported no major complications and showed improvement in snoring and sleepiness in all patients, with an improvement in the IHI according to Sher's criteria of 71.8%. The only negative effect reported is a modest post-operative pain, greater in the case of tonsillectomy.

In 2014 Salamanca et al. [53] proposed a modification of the technique, the Barbed anterior pharyngoplasty, introducing the use of self-locking "hooked" wires (QUill ® knotless tissue closure device, angiotech

Pharmaceutical inc., Vancouver, canada). The technique involves a rectangular incision like that made by Pang, the closest possible to the pterygoid hamulus where the muscle suture is anchored to be fixed to bone structures. Then with a continuous suture the muscular part of the palate is sutured. And then the same procedure is repeated on a submucosal level.

At this point, to further stabilize the palate, a suture is made by anchoring the palate to the posterior nasal spine and bilaterally to the pterygoid hamulus and to the mandibular raphe creating a suspension of the edge of the soft palate and the posterior palatine pillars.

Obtaining at the end of the procedure a palate shortened and projected forward. The only reported side effect was a modest uvular edema and moderate pain for about ten days. Within 4-6 weeks the final fibrosis and consequent stiffening of the palate was obtained.

Barbed Reposition Pharyngoplasty (BRP)

This new technique developed by Vicini et al. [54], arises from the idea of using self-locking wires applied to a technique similar to relocation faringoplasty [51]. It is based on the principle that the palatine pillars and the palate are considered as a tripod and weakening the posterior palatine pillar and moving it forward tends to unbalance the whole system forward increasing the mesopharynx space. The first step consists in tonsillectomy with careful preservation of the mucosa of the anterior and posterior pillars, therefore the lower portion of the palate-pharyngeal muscle is partially incised weakening it. Then a full-thickness mucosa and muscle triangle is removed at the upper lateral edge of the tonsillar loggia to obtain a wider and more squared space at the level of the pharyngeal vestibule. The needle is then introduced at the level of the posterior palatal spine, made to pass completely through the palate in a lateral direction, then around the pterigo-mandibular raphe and is taken out of the bed of the tonsillectomy and then passed through the upper part of the palate muscle pharyngeal making it come out near the mucosa of the posterior pillar, but not crossing it. Then the needle is passed again through the palatopharyngeal muscle and through the raphe by suspending the posterior pillar. By allowing the posterior pillar to be positioned in a more lateral and anterior position, this passage is repeated several times up to the most distal part of the palate-pharyngeal muscle and therefore the thread is passed through the soft palate blocking it.

This technique is currently the most used in our group with excellent results both for snoring and apnea. The only side effect was the pain and the sense of foreign body, which is reduced within a couple of weeks.

Hypopharyngeal Surgery

Hypopharyngeal surgery is basically divided into hyoid surgery and tongue surgery.

Hyoid Surgery

The hyoid surgery consists mainly of the thyro-thyroid disease or suspension of the hyoid. Represents the most reviewed and most documented mode of management of hypopharyngeal collapse, especially on the side walls. The modern surgical procedure, according to Ryley [55] is not very complex, rapid and relatively effective, especially in the range of moderate OSAS even if it is undergoing a progressive decline in recent years as it is considered no longer valid in the management of hypopharyngeal collapses and therefore used only in some selected cases in association with the plastic of the palate.

The indications are:

- Moderate OSAS
- Presence of obstruction at the retrolingual level

A horizontal skin incision of about 3-4 cm is made at an intermediate distance between the inferior edge of the hyoid and upper edge of the thyroid cartilage, possibly at the level of a skin fold. Once the hyoid is identified, a myotomy of the muscles inserted on it is performed, this varies according to the authors. According to the original technique the infraioid muscles are completely detached and the hyoid ligaments are dissected from the lesser cornu, while the suprahyoid musculature is left intact.

In our experience we prefer to dissect both the suprahyoid and subioid muscles, up to the level of the lesser cornu, leaving the stylohyoid ligament intact. In this way we obtain a better mobilization of the hyoid that allows us to overtake the anterior margin of the thyroid cartilage in pexia, but still maintains a good traction on the musculature of the lateral walls of the pharynx which is largely adherent to the great cornu of the Hyoid. This allows the side walls of the pharynx to be in tension and the base of the tongue to advance. At this point the pre-thyroid muscles are separated medially, to allow the identification of the thyroid notch, and the thyroid pexia is performed by 2 points per side with Vicryl n° 1, while in the meantime trying to gently draw forward the iode in the attempt to make them overtake the upper edge of the thyroid cartilage. If the traction is excessive can happen that fractures the hyoid, in these cases it is sufficient to proceed with pexia correctly and usually has no influence on the outcome of the surgery. Normally a small drainage is placed, the muscles above and below the hyoid and all the subcutaneous planes are recovered and then the skin is closed with an intradermal suture.

The surgery does not present any particular post-operative pain, there may be a transient dysphagia which usually resolves in a few days [71]. Rarely, other post-operative complications may occur, such as the most frequent hematoma, seroma, scarring and transient joint distortion. Only Riley assessed the efficacy of the ioidea suspension as a single intervention in the treatment of OSAS, with a 53% success rate.

Tongue Surgery

The tongue surgery is a field that over the years has become increasingly wider, because it is adding numerous techniques ranging from minimally invasive radiofrequency surgery to partial glossectomies. The procedures can be roughly grouped into three categories: tongue reductions, glossopexy and glossectomies.

Tongue Reductions

Most authors perform this procedure by applying radiofrequencies, which represent the single least invasive procedure on hypopharyngeal obstruction and vibration.

The indications are represented by:

- Predominantly lymphatic lingual base hypertrophy
- Simple non-palatal snoring
- Mild to moderate OSAS with predominant retro-lingual obstructive component

It is the only hypopharyngeal procedure that can be performed under local and outpatient anesthesia. Depending on the device used, 8 to 16 applications are used, the application pattern is variable. The main precautions are to avoid repeating the infixion in the same spot and to avoid an excessive duration of the application such as to cause thermal damage to the mucosal level, which creates an important pain and consequent dysphagia for a few days. It is however preferable to have one night of observation after the treatment.

The most severe complication, although not frequent, is the abscess of the base of the tongue [56]. The ulceration of the lingual base mucosa is much more frequent, usually due to too superficial or prolonged application of the electrode.

Glossopexy

The glossopexy are techniques based on the application of devices for containing and anchoring the base of the tongue, aimed at preventing its posterior collapse.

In fact various kits have been developed including the best known is the Repose system (Influ-ENT, USA). It consists of a non-resorbable suture that is passed with two loops around the base of the tongue and then fixed thanks to a screw at the inner edge of the chin [57].

The technique was almost completely abandoned due to the partial results, average success rate of 32.6%, comparable to the less invasive RF.

Another technique is the one developed by Woodson [58] with the ADVANCE system which consists in the surgical positioning of an anchorage system of the midline tissue of the posterior portion of the tongue connected to an anchorage at the level of the adjustable mandibular bone with a flexible tether. But the high failure rate from anchoring in the tissue of the device precluded its clinical use.

Glossectomy

A factor to be carefully evaluated in tongue base surgery is the rich vascular network provided by the lingual artery. According to Vicini et al. [59] the base of the tongue does not offer safe and reproducible landmarks, except for a rich arterial network that approaches the constantly present midline. And theoretically this can be used as an anatomical plane above which there are no large nerves or vessels.

Trans-cervical resection of the base of the tongue was developed in the 1990s by Chabolle et al. [60] when even minimally invasive volumetric reduction techniques were not available. For these reasons this technique has been totally abandoned.

Subsequently, several techniques of transverse oral lingual resection have been proposed.

Woodson and Fujita [61] recommend the excision of the front corner of the resection of a 3 cm side wedge in order to create a defect.

Because of their invasiveness and post-operative morbidity these techniques are considered reserved for patients with severe OSAS who are not compliant with nCPAP therapy. It can be considered an alternative therapeutic option in severe apnea in overweight subjects as an alternative to bimascillary advancement.

Thanks to the emergence of new technologies, some authors have tried to overcome the highly invasive technique. The former were Maturo and Mair [62] using the plasma-mediated bipolar radiofrequency technology (coblator) and then Friedman et al. [63] who developed the submucosal minimally invasive lingual excision (SMILE). This technique involves the prior identification of the course of the lingual arteries with doppler. He then proceeds to a medial incision with a cold blade scalpel, then proceeds with tissue removal with coblator with movements from the top down, paying attention to stay within 1 cm from the median line and medial to the previously marked arteries.

The advent of trans oral robotic surgery (TORS) has allowed the emergence of a further alternative in the management of the lingual base, similar to what happens with oncological surgery.

Lee et al. [64] achieved a 45% success rate in the treatment of severe OSAS with lingual tonsillectomy with TORS and UPPP, with an average AHI reduction from 55.6 to 24.1.

Friedman et al. [65] compared the efficacy of TORS in the management of obstruction of the base of the tongue with that of the coblator and the RF. In none of the 3 groups were major bleeding reported, with similar post-operative pain. The average AHI reductions were 60.5% ± 24.9% for TORS, 37.0% ± 51.6% for the Coblator and 32.0% ± 43.3% for radiofrequency, respectively. Furthermore the authors affirmed the possibility and safety of performing the TORS for the lingual base without the need for tracheotomy.

Vicini et al. [66] with lingual tonsillectomy with TORS obtained a reduction of AHI from 38.3 +/- 23.5 to 20.6 +/- 17.3 with no particular pain-related disorders, difficulty swallowing and no particular complications. Therefore he claims that in case of important hypertrophy of the base of the tongue, minimally invasive techniques are absolutely insufficient and only an adequate removal of tissue can effectively increase the space. Therefore the TORS can be considered in some cases a valid alternative also to the bimascillary advancement in the management of obstructions at the base of the tongue, with a more easily acceptable post-operative course.

HYPOGLOSSAL NERVE STIMULATION

In recent years, thanks to technological progress, the neurostimulation of the lingual musculature during the night is being re-evaluated. In the past the major limitation of these stimulation techniques was the continuous induction of arousals that equally compromised the architecture of sleep [67, 68]. The solution to this problem has been found through selective stimulation of the hypoglossal nerve, which mainly contains efferent motor fibers that give a minimum sensitive afferent feedback.

The musculature of the tongue consists of extrinsic muscles and intrinsic muscles, both groups innervated by the hypoglossal nerve, except the palatoglossus which is innervated by the pharyngeal plexus.

It is above all the stimulation of the genioglossus that has the greatest role, as it represents the major dilator of the VAS, allows the protrusion of the tongue and the tension of the anterior pillars.

The neurostimulator is implanted under general anesthesia, through a small submandibular incision. Then the hypoglossus is exposed inferiorly to the submandibular and above the tendon of the digastric. Once the nerve is isolated, the cuff with the electrodes is placed on the main nerve trunk distal to the branch that innervates the retrusor muscles. This is done thanks to the intraoperative nerve stimulation which allows to identify the correct level to which the neuro-stimulator can be applied based on the muscular response obtained. In the case of neuro stimulators with thoracic sensor, the sensor is tunneled subcutaneously in the ipsilateral infraclavicular space. After 30 days the device is activated and the patient is subjected to a night polysomnography for titration, in order to find the difficult balance between stimulation and tolerance without arousals.

Certal and coll. [69] in a recent review they compared the effectiveness of existing systems, highlighting an improvement in the AHI, the overall reduction in the AHI was 54% at 3 months, 57% at 6 months, and 50% at 12 months.

None of the analyzed studies reported serious side effects, but in 4.5% of patients it was necessary to resort to explanting the device. The defined indications were BMI $\leq$ 32 kg/m2, AHI between 20 and 50 without complete concentric collapse at the level of the soft palate, patients with bulky tongues reported better results. They noted some technical differences in particular with regard to the multi-electrode system that only targets the desired parts of the hypoglossal nerve, allowing a high degree of specificity. The targeted activation of the genioglossus muscle avoids the need to synchronize stimulation with the respiratory cycle and can reduce some of the costs related to surgical time.

Laringeal Surgery

Although the most frequent obstruction sites are those in the retropalatal and retrolingual level, the larynx can also contribute to the genesis of OSAS. It is essential to distinguish pediatric forms from those of adults, as in the former the main causes of obstruction are laryngomalacia, malformations and only rarely from neoformations, neoplasms or laryngeal paralysis. While in the adult the causes are specularly opposite.

Laryngeal obstruction plays a minor role in the adult compared to the child in the determinism of the OSAS.

Possible anatomo-functional conditions to be treated:

1. laryngeal diplegia;
2. laryngeal monoplegia;
3. floppy epiglottis;
4. tumors;
5. post radiotherapy larynx;
6. post-reconstructive neolaringe;
7. acquired laryngomalacia (laryngeal trauma, sarcoidosis, acromegaly, etc.);
8. stridor from MSA;

In the case of floppy epiglottis, a partial resection is indicated, usually V or horizontal in the free part associated with a shortening of the glosso-epiglottic ligament [70].

It is essential to use sleep-endoscopy in cases with suspected laryngeal obstruction, since CPAP therapy is not possible in the case of floppy epiglottis because positive pressure air presses the epiglottis against the laryngeal vestibule as if it were a lid, worsening the situation [72]. In these cases, there is no alternative to surgery. The decisive criterion is not the size of the epiglottis but its rigidity. In the case of very flaccid epiglottids, a partial resection should be considered, but if the cause of the prolapse is related to the posterior thrust operated by the base of the tongue, it is on this that one must act with a volumetric reduction or with hyoid advancement.

FACIAL SKELETON SURGERY

Unlike the interventions described above, it acts on the container and not on the content, allowing an extension of the UA. It is very effective being comparable to CPAP but it is also very invasive and has relevant anatomical and aesthetic modifications.

There are numerous groups of different procedures reviewed on the facial skeleton:

1. Advancement of the isolated genioglossus muscle or integrated with other procedures: This procedure is practiced entirely orally through an incision on the gingival mucosa, creating an advancement of the base of the tongue.

   It represents an invasive technique, with a high risk of complications, it has been replaced by most groups by less invasive techniques such as RF of the base of the tongue.
2. Isolated mandibular advancements.
3. Maxillo-mandibular advancements: Designed by Kuo et al. [73], today it is surgery with the greatest success rate after tracheotomy. But it is a complex and invasive intervention with high morbidity and complications, and considerable aesthetic consequences. It allows the simultaneous dilation of all the rhino-hypo-pharyngeal

structures thanks to the increase of the volumes of the UA with tensioning of the lateral walls of the pharynx and advancement of the soft palate and the base of the tongue. It is one of the few surgical procedures that does not require an oropharyngeal time on the palate. Many studies have shown the effectiveness of maxillo-mandibular progress compared with CPAP. In a meta-analysis and systematic review of the literature Holty et al. [74] showed an average reduction in the AHI from 63.9/h to 9.5/h.

4. Rapid expansions of the upper jaw.
5. Anterior and transverse maxillary osteodistraction procedures: It is used when the advance must be greater than 10 mm or in children, as progressive progression reduces the risk of alveolar nerve injury. The procedure involves osteotomies similar to AMM, but these are mobilized only progressively (usually 1 mm per day) after a few days under the guidance of distractors. Thus non-mineralized tissue fills the osteotomy gap which is slowly lengthening and after the end of distraction it will turn into bone during the consolidation period. Since there are multidirectional distractors, it is possible to correct the distraction vector during treatment.

TRACHEAL SURGERY

Tracheotomy was the first effective treatment on OSAS and still remains the last but most certain resource [75].

It is indicated in some cases

1. In urgency: in case of newborns with severe respiratory distress, also due to VAS malformations, following surgical complications.
2. Pending: in the presence of laryngomalacia with severe OSAS, or in children with facial cranial anomalies awaiting surgery
3. Alternatively; to CPAP or other types of surgery especially in the case of patients with morbid obesity.

4. In recovery of techniques, however indicated in the most serious cases (advancement of bilaxel or Chabolle) did not go well.

The success rate is close to 100%, but in patients with cardiopulmonary decompensation the trachestomy reduces drastically but does not eliminate the OSAS problem probably due to the persistence of central events, and in some cases due to the occlusion of the ostomy by the tissue exuberant fat.

In adult patients in the rare cases in which the tracheotomy is a procedure of choice in our experience, it is preferable to perform a so-called "skin lined" technique [76] in which the edges of the tracheostoma are covered laterally and upper-inferiorly by two flaps of tracheal mucosa. This technique allows to obtain a more stable tracheostoma, which does not undergo the formation of granulation tissue and allows the eventual daily occlusion.

Bariatric Surgery

Bariatric surgery is indicated for significant weight loss in patients with BMI> 40 kg/m2 or in those with BMI ≥ 35 kg/m2 but with important comorbidities and where dietary recommendations were not successful. This therapy should be implemented in conjunction with ventilatory therapy, and the severity of the OSAS should be re-evaluated following weight loss. A reduction in OSAS has been reported, following weight loss after two years of bariatric surgery of 40% [77].

References

[1] American Academy of Sleep Medicine. *Obstructive Sleep Apnea.* 2008.

[2] *AAO-HNS Treatment of Obstructive Sleep Apnea* http://www.entnet.org/content/treatment-obstructive-sleep-apnea#

[3] American Sleep Apnea Association website. *OSA treatment options.* 2012.

[4] Cahali MB. Lateral pharyngoplasty: A new treatment for obstructive sleep apnea hypopnea syndrome. *Laryngoscope.* 2003 Nov;113(11):1961-8.

[5] Pang KP, Woodson BT. Expansion sphincter pharyngoplasty: a new technique for the treatment of obstructive sleep apnea. *Otolaryngol Head Neck Surg.* 2007 Jul;137(1):110-4.

[6] Vicini C, Hendawy E, Campanini A, Eesa M, Bahgat A, AlGhamdi S, Meccariello G, DeVito A, Montevecchi F, Mantovani M. Barbed reposition pharyngoplasty (BRP) for OSAHS: a feasibility, safety, efficacy and teachability pilot study. "We are onthe giant's shoulders". *Eur Arch Otorhinolaryngol.* 2015 Apr 12.

[7] Rubin AH, Eliaschar I, Joachim Z, Alroy G, Lavie P. Effects of nasal surgery and tonsillectomy on sleep apnea. *Bull Eur Physiopathol Respir* 1983; 19: 612–615.

[8] Modica DM, Marchese D, Lorusso F, Speciale R, Saraniti C, Gallina S. Functional Nasal Surgery and Use of CPAP in OSAS Patients: Our Experience. *Indian J Otolaryngol Head Neck Surg.* 2018 Dec;70(4):559-565.

[9] Friedman M, Tanyeri H, Lim JW, Landsberg R, Vaidyanathan K, Caldarelli D. Effect of improved nasal breathing on obstructive sleep apnea. *Otolaryngol Head Neck Surg* 2000; 122: 71–74.

[10] Dorn M, Pirsig W, Verse T. Management of patients with severe obstructive sleep apnea following rhinosurgical interventions. A pilot study [in German]. *HNO* 2001; 49: 642–645.

[11] Lorusso F, Martines F, Mistretta A, Alagna E, Modica Dm, Dispenza F, Gallina S. Effects of adenotonsillectomy on neurocognitive and behavioural function in pediatric obstructive sleep apnea syndrome. *B-ENT*, 2018, 14, 113-118.

[12] Hibbert J, Stell P. Adenoidectomy. An evaluation of the indications. *Arch Dis Child* 1978; 53: 910–911.

[13] Maw AR, Jeans WD, Cable HR. Adenoidectomy. A prospective study to show clinical and radiological changes two years after operation. *J Laryngol Otol* 1983; 97: 511–518.

[14] Nieminen P, Tolonen U, Löppönen H. Snoring and obstructive sleep apnea in children. A 6-month follow-up study. *Arch Otolaryngol Head Neck Surg* 2000; 126: 481–486.

[15] Guidelines in roncosurgery ENT - Italian Society of Otorhinolaryngology and Head and Neck Surgery – Topics of Acta Otorhinolaryngologica Italica 2007.

[16] Arens R, McDonough JM, Costarino AT, et al. Magnetic resonance imaging of the upper airway structure of children with obstructive sleep apnea syndrome. *Am J Respir Crit Care Med.* 2001;164:698–703.

[17] Shintani T, Asakura K, Kataura A. Adenotonsillar hypertrophy and skeletal morphology of children with obstructive sleep apnea syndrome. *Acta Otolaryngol Suppl.* 1996;523:222–4.

[18] Kara CO, Ergin H, Kocak G, Kilic I, Yurdakul M. Prevalence of tonsillar hypertrophy and associated oropharyngeal symptoms in primary school children in Denizli, Turkey. *Int J Pediatr Otorhinolaryngol.* 2002;66:175–9.

[19] Hörmann K, Verse T. Surgery for Sleep-Disordered Breathing. Springer-Verlag Berlin Heidelberg 2005.

[20] Lorusso F, Gallina S, Modica DM, Di Salvo N, Riggio F. Bipolar Quantum Molecular Resonance versus Blunt Dissection tonsillectomy. *B-ENT.* 2015;11(2):101-8.

[21] Hilton M. Tonsillectomy technique-tradition versus technology. *Lancet.* 2004;364:642-3.

[22] Hultcrantz E, Linder A, Markström A. Tonsillectomy or tonsillotomy? A randomized study comparing postoperative pain and long-term effects. *Int J Pediatr Otorhinolaryngol* 1999; 51: 171–176.

[23] Whinney DJ, Williamson PA, Bicknell PG. Punctate diathermy of the soft palate: a new approach in the surgical management of snoring. *J Laryngol Otol* 1995; 109: 849–852.

[24] Sundaram S, Bridgman SA, Lim J, Lasserson TJ. Surgery for obstructive sleep apnoea. *Cochrane Database Syst Rev.* 2005 Oct 19;(4):CD001004. Review.

[25] *SNLG Appropriatezza e sicurezza degli interventi di tonsillectomia e/o adenoidectomia.* 2008.http://www.snlg-iss.it/lgn.

[26] Baugh RF, Archer SM, Mitchell RB, Rosenfeld RM, Amin R, Burns JJ, Darrow DH, Giordano T, Litman RS, Li KK, Mannix ME, Schwartz RH, Setzen G, Wald ER, Wall E, Sandberg G, Patel MM; American Academy of Otolaryngology-Head and Neck Surgery Foundation. Clinical practice guideline: Tonsillectomy in children. *Otolaryngol Head Neck Surg.* 2011 Jan;144(1 Suppl):S1-30.

[27] Lescanne E, Chiron B, Constant I, Couloigner V, Fauroux B, Hassani Y, Jouffroy L, Lesage V, Mondain M, Nowak C, Orliaguet G, Viot A; French Society of ENT (SFORL); French Association for Ambulatory Surgery (AFCA); French Society for Anaesthesia, Intensive Care (SFAR). Pediatric tonsillectomy: clinical practice guidelines. *Eur Ann Otorhinolaryngol Head Neck Dis.* 2012 Oct;129(5):264-71.

[28] Brietzke S, Gallagher D, The effectiveness of tonsillectomy and adenoidectomy in the treatment of pediatric obstructive sleep apnea/hypopnea syndrome: A meta-analysis. *Otolaryngol Head Neck Surg,* 134(6), 979-984, 2006.

[29] Tzifa KT, Shehab ZP, Robin PE. The relation between tonsillectomy and snoring. *Clin Otolaryngol* 1998; 23: 148–151.

[30] Nelson LM. Radiofrequency treatment for obstructive tonsillar hypertrophy. *Arch Otolaryngol Head Neck Surg* 2000; 126: 736–740.

[31] Mortimore IL, Bradley PA, Murray JA, Douglas NJ. Uvulopalatopharyngoplasty may compromise nasal CPAP therapy in sleep apnea syndrome. *Am J Respir Crit Care Med* 1996; 154:1759–1762.

[32] Cahali MB. Lateral pharyngoplasty: a new treatment for obstructive sleep apnea hypopnea syndrome. *Laryngoscope.* 2003 Nov;113(11):1961-8.

[33] Brietzke SE, Mair EA. Injection snoreplasty: how to treat snoring without all the pain and expense. *Otolaryngol Head Neck Surg* 2001; 124: 503–510.

[34] Choi JH, Kim SN, Cho JH. Efficacy of the Pillar implant in the treatment of snoring and mild-to-moderate obstructive sleep apnea: a meta-analysis. *Laryngoscope.* 2013 Jan; 123(1):269-76.

[35] Hur J. A new treatment for snoring: sling snoreplasty with a permanent thread. *Acta otolaryngol* 2008;128:1381-4.

[36] Mantovani M, Minetti A, Torretta S, Pincherle A, Tassone G, Pignataro L. The velo-uvulo-pharyngeal lift or "roman blinds" technique for treatment of snoring: A preliminary report. *Acta Otorhinolaryngol Ital.* 2012 Feb;32(1):48-53.

[37] Mantovani M, Minetti A, Torretta S, Pincherle A, Tassone G, Pignataro L. The "Barbed Roman Blinds" technique: a step forward. *Acta Otorhinolaryngol Ital.* 2013 Apr;33(2):128.

[38] Haavisto L, Suonpaa J. Complications of uvulopalatoplasty. *Clin Otolaryngol* 1994; 19: 243–247.

[39] Katsantonis GP, Friedman WH, Krebs FJ, Walsh JK. Nasopharyngeal complications following uvulopalatopharyngoplasty. *Laryngoscope* 1987; 97: 309–314.

[40] Mortimore IL, Bradley PA, Murray JA, Douglas NJ. Uvulopalatopharyngoplasty may compromise nasal CPAP therapy in sleep apnea syndrome. *Am J Respir Crit Care Med* 1996; 154:1759–1762.

[41] Hassid S, Afrapoli AH, Decaaestecker C, Cho- ufani G. UPPP for snoring: long-term results and patient satisfaction. *Acta Otorhinolaryngol Belg* 2002; 56: 157–162.

[42] Sher AE, Schechtman KB, Piccirillo JF. The efficacy of surgical modifications of the upper airway in adults with obstructive sleep apnea syndrome. *Sleep* 1996; 19: 156–177.

[43] Aurora RN, Casey KR, Kristo D, et al. Practice parameters for the surgical modifications of the upper airway for obstructive sleep apnea in adults. *Sleep.* 2010a;33(10):1408-1413.

[44] Carenfelt C. Laser uvulopalatopharyngoplasty in treatment of habitual snoring. *Ann Otol Rhinol Laryngol* 1991; 100: 451–454.

[45] Kamami YV. Laser CO2 for snoring: preliminary results. *Acta Otorhinolaryngol Belg* 1990; 44:451–456.

[46] Morar P, Nandapalan V, Lesser THJ, Swift AC. Mucosal-strip/uvulectomy by the CO2 laser as a method of treating simple snoring. *Clin Oto-laryngol* 1995; 20: 308–311.

[47] Astor FC, Hanft KL, Benson C, Amaranath A. Analysis of short-term outcome after office-based laser-assisted uvulopalatoplasty. *Otolaryngol Head Neck Surg* 1998; 118: 478–480.

[48] Mesti JJ, Cahali MB. Evolution of swallowing in lateral pharyngoplasty with stylopharyngeal muscle preservation. *Braz J Otorhinolaryngol.* 2012 Dec;78(6):51-5.

[49] Pang KP, Woodson BT. Expansion sphincter pharyngoplasty: a new technique for the treatment of obstructive sleep apnea. *Otolaryngol Head Neck Surg.* 2007 Jul;137(1):110-4.

[50] Lorusso F, Dispenza F, Modica DM, Gallina S. The Role of Modified Expansion Sphincter Pharyngoplasty in Multilevel Obstructive Sleep Apnea Syndrome Surgery. *Int Arch Otorhinolaryngol.* 2018 Oct;22(4):432-436.

[51] Li HY, Lee LA (2009) Relocation pharyngoplasty for obstructive sleep apnea. *Laryngoscope* 119:2472–2477.

[52] Pang KP, Tan R, Puraviappan P, Terris DJ. Anterior palatoplasty for the treatment of OSA: three-year results. *Otolaryngol Head Neck Surg.* 2009 Aug;141(2):253-6.

[53] Salamanca F, Costantini F, Mantovani M, Bianchi A, Amaina T, Colombo E, Zibordi F. Barbed anterior pharyngoplasty: an evolution of anterior palatoplasty. *Acta Otorhinolaryngol Ital.* 2014 Dec;34(6):434-438. Review.

[54] Vicini C, Hendawy E, Campanini A, Eesa M, Bahgat A, AlGhamdi S, Meccariello G, DeVito A, Montevecchi F, Mantovani M. Barbed reposition pharyngoplasty (BRP) for OSAHS: a feasibility, safety, efficacy and teachability pilot study. "We are onthe giant's shoulders". *Eur Arch Otorhinolaryngol.* 2015 Apr 12.

[55] Riley RW, Powell NB, Guilleminault C. Obstructive sleep apnea and the hyoid: a revised surgical procedure. *Otolaryngol Head Neck Surg* 1994; 111: 717–721.

[56] Pazos G, Mair EA. Complications of radiofrequency ablation in the treatment of sleep-disordered breathing. Otolaryngol Head Neck Surg 2001; 125: 462–466.

[57] DeRowe A, Günther E, Fibbi A, Lehtimaki K, Vahatalo K, Maurer J, Ophir D. Tongue-base suspension with a soft tissue-to-bone anchor for obstructive sleep apnea: preliminary clinical results of a new minimally invasive technique. *Otolaryngol Head Neck Surg* 2000; 122; 100–103.

[58] Multicenter study of a novel adjustable tongue-advancement device for obstructive sleep apnea. Woodson BT, Steward DL, Mickelson S, Huntley T, Goldberg A. *Otolaryngol Head Neck Surg.* 2010 Oct;143(4):585-90. doi: 10.1016/j.otohns.2010.06.902.

[59] Transoral robotic surgery of the tongue base in obstructive sleep Apnea Hypopnea syndrome Anatomic considerations and clinical experience.

[60] Chabolle F, Wagner I, Blumen M, Séquert C, Fleury B, de Dieuleveult T. Tongue base reduction with hyoepiglottoplasty: A treatment for severe obstructive sleep apnea. Laryngoscope 1999; 109:1273–1280

[61] Woodson BT, Fujita S. Clinical experience with lingualplasty as part of the treatment of severe obstructive sleep apnea. *Otolaryngol Head Neck Surg* 1992; 107: 40–48.

[62] Maturo SC, Mair EA. Submucosal minimally invasive lingual excision: An effective, novel surgery for pediatric tongue base reduction. *Ann Otol Rhinol Laryngol* 2006; 115:624–30.

[63] Friedman M, Soans R, Gurpinar B, Lin HC, Joseph N. Evaluation of submucosal minimally invasive lingual excision technique for treatment of obstructive sleep apnea/hypopnea syndrome. *Otolaryngol Head Neck Surg.* 2008 Sep;139(3):378-84.

[64] Lee JM, Weinstein GS, O'Malley BW Jr, Thaler ER. Transoral robot-assisted lingual tonsillectomy and uvulopalatopharyngoplasty

for obstructive sleep apnea. *Ann Otol Rhinol Laryngol.* 2012 Oct;121(10):635-9.

[65] Friedman M, Hamilton C, Samuelson CG, et al. Transoral robotic glossectomy for the treatment of obstructive sleep apnea-hypopnea syndrome. *Otolaryngol Head Neck Surg.* 2012 May;146(5):854-62.

[66] Vicini C, Dallan I, Canzi P, et al. Transoral robotic tongue base resection in obstructive sleep apnoea-hypopnoea syndrome: a preliminary report. *ORL J Otorhinolaryngol Relat Spec.* 2010;72(1):22-7. Epub 2010 Feb 18.

[67] REDLINE S. Genetics of obstructive sleep apnea. In: KRYGER MH, ROTH T, DEMENT WC, eds. *Principles and Practice of Sleep Medicine.* Philadelphia: Elsevier Saunders, 2005:1013–1022.

[68] Smith PL, Eisele DW, Podszus T, et al. Electrical stimulation of upper airway musculature. *Sleep* 1996;19:S284-7.

[69] Certal VF, Zaghi S, Riaz M, Vieira AS, Pinheiro CT, Kushida C, Capasso R, Camacho M. Hypoglossal nerve stimulation in the treatment of obstructive sleep apnea: A systematic review and meta-analysis. *Laryngoscope.* 2014 Nov 12.

[70] Golz A, Goldenberg D, Netzer A, Westerman ST, Joachims HZ. Epiglottic carcinoma presenting as obstructive sleep apnea. *J Otolaryngol* 2001; 30: 58–59.

[71] Lorusso F, Dispenza F, Martinciglio G, Messina A, Battaglia A, Gallina S. Postural changes in patients undergoing hyoid surgery for osas. *Euromediterranean biomedical journal* 2017, 12 (29) 140–143 (formerly: capsula eburnea).

[72] Verse T, Pirsig W. Age-related changes in the epiglottis causing failure of nasal continuous positive airway pressure therapy. *J Laryngol Otol* 1999; 113: 1022–1025.

[73] Kuo PC, West RA, Bloomquist DS, McNeil RW. The effect of mandibular osteotomy in three patients with hypersomnia sleep apnea. *Oral Surg Oral Med Oral Path* 1979; 48: 385–392.

[74] Holty JE, Guilleminault C. Maxillomandibular advancement for the treatment of obstructive sleep apnea: a systematic review and meta-analysis. *Sleep Med Rev.* 2010 Oct; 14(5):287-97.

[75] Kuhlo W, Doll E, Franck MC. Successful management of Pickwickian syndrome using long-term tracheostomy [in German]. *Dtsch Med Wschr* 1969; 94: 1286–1290.

[76] Fee WE Jr, Ward PH. Permanent tracheostomy: A new surgical technique. *Ann Otol Rhinol Laryngol.* 1977 Sep-Oct;86(5 Pt 1): 635-8.

[77] Mechanick JI, Kushner RF, Sugerman HJ, Gonzalez-Campoy JM, Collazo-Clavell ML, Guven S, Spitz AF, Apovian CM, Livingston EH, Brolin R, Sarwer DB, Anderson WA, Dixon J. American Association of Clinical Endocrinologists, The Obesity Society, and American Society for Metabolic & Bariatric Surgery Medical guidelines for clinical practice for the perioperative nutritional, metabolic, and nonsurgical support of the bariatric surgery patient. *Endocr Pract.* 2008 Jul-Aug; 14.

In: New Research on Sleep …
Editor: Olivier Ratté
ISBN: 978-1-53616-882-2

Chapter 9

The Role of Drug-Induced Sleep/Sedation Endoscopy (DISE) in the Detection of OSAHS

A. Mistretta, MD, A. Battaglia, MD, S. Gallina **[*]**
and F. Lorusso **[≠]*****, MD***
Unit of Otolaringology, Department of Experimental Biomedicine and Clinical Neurosciences, Polyclinic University Hospital "Paolo Giaccone," University of Palermo, Palermo, Italy

Abstract

Dynamic airway study during sleep is a clinical challenge in OSAS, in order to target obstruction sites as well as possible. Drug-induced sleep/sedation endoscopy (DISE) was first described by Croft and Pringle in 1991.

According to the "European Position Paper On Drug Induced Sedation Endoscopy (DISE)," written in 2014 by a group of experts of DISE, this exam should be performed in patients affected by disturbing

---

* Professor.
≠ Corresponding Author's E-mail: dott.francescolorusso@gmail.com.

snoring and OSAHS, in whom non-CPAP therapy is considered. DISE may be also be performed in patients who have failed or don't tolerate CPAP therapy.

Moreover, it can be useful to describe why a previous surgery has failed, and how to solve it.

Absolute contraindications to DISE are ASA 4, pregnancy, and patients with an allergy to DISE drugs. Relative contraindications may include morbid obesity.

Talking about drugs to induce sleep, *propofol* and *midazolam* are the most commonly used to perform DISE; *dexmedetomidine* has demonstrated to be suitable as sedative agent too, so it could be used much more in the future.

ENT performing DISE can classify obstruction patterns in several ways, for example with NOHL (Nose, Oropharynx, Hypopharynx and Larynx) or VOTE (Velum, Oropharyngeal wall, Tongue Base, Epiglottis) classifications.

Odontologists can test mandibular advancement devices (MAD) in patients during DISE, in order to set them in the most effective shape to prevent sleep apneas/ hypopneas.

DISE is nowadays a relatively simple way to explore obstruction sites during induced sleep and, finally, to give the most precise indication for surgery (technique and timing); of course it has to be improved in a lot of features: it should be cheaper, quicker, and it should be performed in an almost "natural" sleep.

INTRODUCTION

Dynamic airway study during sleep is a clinical challenge in OSAS, in order to target obstruction sites as well as possible. This exam has been called during time in different ways. It was first described by Croft and Pringle in 1991 [1] as sleep nasendoscopy, abbreviated SNE. Other names used are: sleep endoscopy [2, 3], video sleep nasendoscopy [4], drug-induced sleep endoscopy [5, 6] and fiber-optic sleep endoscopy [7]. According to the Update of the European Position Paper On Drug-Induced Sleep Endoscopy (Dise) of 2017, the most appropriate name is Drug-induced sleep Endoscopy, using "sleep" instead of "sedation"[8].

In 1978 Borowiecki [9] formerly made an endoscopy of upper airway system during physiological sleep, in order to explain how apneas were generated. Pharyngeal airway during sleep was observed with help of fibro-optic flexible bronchoscope and cineradiography in 10 adult patients with Hypersomnia Sleep-Apnea (HSA) syndrome. This procedure was very difficult, long and expensive to make, but suggested that muscles of velopharyngeal sphincter and tongue were mainly responsible for apneas.

In 1991 Croft and Pringle [1] presented the technique of "sleep nasendoscopy" to visualize directly the site or sites of obstruction in a sleeping patient. Their study showed that there were patients with obstructive sleep apnoea syndrome (OSAS) in whom the only site of pharyngeal obstruction was at the velopharynx, so this was the surgical site to treat. For many other OSAS patients in whom obstruction was multisegmental, this exam explained poor results of UVPP and was thought to be a good skill to avoid unnecessary or uncomplete surgery.

In 2014 a group of expert on OSAS and sleep endoscopy (Vicini C, Vanderveken OM, Sorrenti G, Piccin O, Montevecchi F, Maurer J, Kotecha BT, Hohenhorst W, Hamas E, De Vries, Campanini A, Braghiroli A, Bosi M, Vanni A, Llatas MC, De Vito A) met and wrote the "European position paper on drug-induced sedation endoscopy (DISE)" [10]. It has been a first attempt to create a sort of Guidelines about this procedure.

INDICATIONS AND CONTRAINDICATIONS

DISE should be performed in selected patients in whom additional information concerning the dynamics of the UA (sites and patterns) are required. It is useful in case of alternative treatment rather than CPAP, such as upper airway surgery (UAS), oral appliance therapy (OAT) therapy, positional therapy (PT) or a combination of them [11-13],. It can be applied in patients who underwent an unsuccessful treatment, to improve understanding of the anatomical basis for surgical, MAD, or PAP (positive airway pressure) failure. For example, it can be performed with and without simultaneous OAT and PAP application, in order to check therapy improvements and failures [14, 15]. DISE may be even performed in patients who encounter difficulties in tolerating CPAP, trying to highlight reasons for this difficulty [8].

The application of DISE, plus the correct diagnosis obtained by PSG, and a specific "Upper Airways" examination, assist in predicting surgical outcomes [16, 17].

How to Perform DISE

DISE should be performed in patients with acceptable overall anesthetic risk profile. Absolute contraindications are ASA 4 and pregnancy, and allergy to DISE sedative agents. Relative contraindications may include morbid obesity [8].

Before executing DISE, it is mandatory to do types 1, 2, or 3 sleep studies according to American Academy of Sleep Medicine (AASM) clinical and endoscopic awake UA examination, and clinical presedation assessment. The exam should be done in any safe clinical setting with standard anaesthetic equipment. Instruments needed are: standard anaesthesiological monitoring [oxygen saturation ($SatO_2$), electrocardiogram (ECG), blood pressure (BP)] and flexible endoscope. An infusion pump or a target-controlled infusion (TCI) if the drug to be used is propofol, and electroencephalogram (EEG)-derived indices are also required, but aren't mandatory. Bispectral (BIS) index or cerebral state index (CSI), entropy, as well as polygraphic realtime monitoring are useful to assess the depth of sedation and anesthesia [8].

Preparatory measures such as nasal decongestion, nasal local anesthesia, and antisecretory drugs can potentially interact with UA and breathing control and therefore have to be used with caution. Instead of the latter, a surgical aspirator can be very useful if hypersalivation occurs [18].

According to PSG results, DISE should be performed not only in supine position but also in non-supine, with or without pillow(s) according to the patient's usual sleep habit. It's better starting the exam in "worst sleeping position" [19]. Changing head position, instead of all body position, can be reliable too, but further studies have to be done about it.

Trans-oral fiber-optic endoscopy in selected patients can help establishing the degree of tongue retraction and position. In addition, if

OAT therapy is considered, the Oral Appliance can be tested and titrated during DISE. *George Gauge* appliance, gradually advancing the jaw from 70-80% until its maximum, shows which is the minimum effective advancement obtainable with OA. It's better making the patient wear the OA before starting the sedation, in order not to disturb his/her sleep [20, 21].

Drugs

The most used drugs (for sedation) to perform DISE are midazolam and propofol, as single agents or together. Some authors combine them with remifentanil or ketamine. Another drug that can be used is Dexmedetomidine, an alpha 2 adrenergic drug that produces sedation plus analgesia by inhibiting the locus ceruleus. A review of 2013 compared the efficacy of Propofol vs Dexmedetomidine among 220 studies, pointing out how they're both effective. Dexmedetomidine ensures cardiopulmonary system stability; propofol has a rapid onset and half-life [22].

According to the Position Paper [8] the ideal observation window lasts at least two cycles or one minute but it may take longer both for each segment of UA and during the maneuvers. A cycle is a complete and stable sequence of snoring–obstructing hypopnea/apnea–oxygen desaturation–breathing with good observation of levels.

If BIS is available, it should be between 80 - 60 during the procedure, obtaining a medium-sedation level status, consisting of loss of response to verbal stimulation at a normal volume [23].

Classification

According to the 2017 Update of European Position Paper on DISE [10], VOTE classification [24] is the one that should be adopted. Authors suggest the possibility of adding comments (e.g., anatomical structures involved in the obstruction) for each level. They chose this one because it's a good compromise between the most used ones; general agreement was considered of higher importance than including all possible and rare forms and exceptions in a standardized classification.

In VOTE Classification

Structures considered are:

- ✓ Velum,
- ✓ Oropharynx lateral walls,
- ✓ Tongue base,
- ✓ Epiglottis.

The degrees of severity are:

- ✓ none,
- ✓ partial,
- ✓ complete.

Possible configurations are:

- ✓ antero-posterior,
- ✓ lateral,
- ✓ concentric.

It's necessary to check the localization of the tip of the endoscope to score the obstruction: at the level of the choanae to assess the soft palate, at the level of the margin of the soft palate to assess the oropharynx, and just above the level of the tongue base to assess the tongue base and the epiglottis.

Conclusion

A review of 2017 [25] underlined how DISE is now widely used and although its value for diagnosis and treatment of sleep-disordered breathing could not yet be demonstrated for all non-CPAP therapies, it may be used in the future as a predictive examination for mandibular advancement devices and respiration-synchronous neurostimulation of the hypoglossal nerve.

The "ideal DISE" should be cheap, easy and rapid to perform; it should be done during spontaneous sleep. These goals are very difficult to achieve. Of course trying to create a "standard exam" among all the possibilities that DISE includes, is one of the most achievable targets at the moment, and it requests further studies.

References

[1] Croft CB, Pringle M (1991) Sleep nasendoscopy: a technique of assessment in snoring and obstructive sleep apnoea. *Clin. Otolaryngol. Allied Sci.* 16:504–509.

[2] Abdullah VJ, Lee DLY, Ha SCN, van Hasselt CA (2013) Sleep endoscopy with midazolam: sedation level evaluation with bispectral analysis. *Otolaryngol. Head Neck Surg.* 148:331–337. doi: 10.1177/0194599812464865.

[3] Bachar G, Feinmesser R, Shpitzer T, et al., (2008) Laryngeal and hypopharyngeal obstruction in sleep disordered breathing patients, evaluated by sleep endoscopy. *Eur. Arch. Otorhinolaryngol.* 265:1397–1402. doi: 10.1007/s00405-008-0637-5.

[4] Abdullah VJ, Wing YK, van Hasselt C a. (2003) Video sleep nasendoscopy: the Hong Kong experience. *Otolaryngol. Clin. North Am.* 36:461–471, vi. doi: 10.1016/S0030-6665(02)00176-7.

[5] Kezirian EJ (2006) Drug-induced sleep endoscopy. *Oper. Tech. Otolaryngol. - Head Neck Surg.* 17:230–232. doi: 10.1016/j.otot.2006.10.005.

[6] Hohenhorst W, Ravesloot MJL, Kezirian EJ, de Vries N (2012) Drug-induced sleep endoscopy in adults with sleep-disordered breathing: Technique and the VOTE Classification system. *Oper. Tech. Otolaryngol.* 23:11–18. doi: 10.1016/j.otot.2011.06.001.

[7] Fishman G, Zemel M, DeRowe A, et al., (2013) Fiber-optic sleep endoscopy in children with persistent obstructive sleep apnea: inter-observer correlation and comparison with awake endoscopy. *Int. J. Pediatr. Otorhinolaryngol.* 77:752–755. doi: 10.1016/j.ijporl.2013.02.002.

[8] De Vito Andrea, Marina Carrasco Llatas, Madeline Ravensloot, Bhik Kotecha, Nico De Vries, Evert Hamans, Joachim Maurer, Marcello Bosi, Marc Blumen, Clemens Heiser, et al. European position paper on drug-induced sleep endoscopy (DISE): 2017 update. *Clin. Otolaryngol.* 2018 Aug 22 Published online 2018 Aug 22. doi: 10.1111/coa.13213.

[9] Borowiecki B., C. P. Pollak, E. D. Weitzman, S. Rakoff, J. Imperato. Fibro-optic study of pharyngeal airway during sleep in patients with hypersomnia obstructive sleep-apnea syndrome. *Laryngoscope.* 1978 Aug; 88(8 Pt 1): 1310–1313. doi: 10.1288/00005537-197808000-00012).

[10] De Vito A, Carrasco Llatas M, Vanni A, et al., (2014) European position paper on drug-induced sedation endoscopy (DISE). *Sleep Breath* 18:453–65. doi: 10.1007/s11325-014-0989-6.

[11] Vanderveken OM (2013) Drug-induced sleep endoscopy (DISE) for non-CPAP treatment selection in patients with sleep-disordered breathing. *Sleep Breath* 17:13–14. doi: 10.1007/s11325-012-0671-9.

[12] Modica DM, Marchese D, Lorusso F, Speciale R, Saraniti C, Gallina S. Functional Nasal Surgery and Use of CPAP in OSAS Patients: Our Experience. *Indian J. Otolaryngol. Head Neck Surg.* 2018 Dec;70(4): 559-565.

[13] Lorusso F, Dispenza F, Modica DM, Gallina S. The Role of Modified Expansion Sphincter Pharyngoplasty in Multilevel Obstructive Sleep Apnea Syndrome Surgery. *Int. Arch. Otorhinolaryngol.* 2018 Oct;22(4):432-436.

[14] Kent DT, Rogers R, Soose RJ. Drug-Induced Sedation Endoscopy in the Evaluation of OSA Patients with Incomplete Oral Appliance Therapy Response. *Otolaryngol. Head Neck Surg*. 2015; 153: 302-7).

[15] Civelek S, Emre IE, Dizdar D, et al., (2012) Comparison of conventional continuous positive airway pressure to continuous positive airway pressure titration performed with sleep endoscopy. *Laryngoscope* 122:691–695. doi: 10.1002/lary.22494.

[16] Koutsourelakis I, Safiruddin F, Ravesloot M, Zakynthinos S, De Vries N. (2012) Surgery for obstructive sleep apnea: sleep endoscopy determinants of outcome. *Laryngoscope* 122(11):2587–91.

[17] Hsu Y-S, Jacobowitz O. (2017). Does Sleep Endoscopy Staging Pattern Correlate with Outcome of Advanced Palatopharyngoplasty for Moderate to Severe Obstructive Sleep Apnea? *J. Clin. Sleep Med.*

[18] Doherty LS, Nolan P, McNicholas WT (2005) Effects of topical anesthesia on upper airway resistance during wake-sleep transitions. *J. Appl. Physiol.* 99:549–555. doi: 10.1152/japplphysiol.01221.2004.

[19] Lee CH, Kim DK, Kim SY, et al., (2015) Changes in site of obstruction in obstructive sleep apnea patients according to sleep position: A DISE study. *Laryngoscope* 125:248–54. doi: 10.1002/lary.24825.

[20] American Academy of Sleep Medicine. Practice parameters for the treatment of snoring and obstructive sleep apnea with oral appliances. *Sleep* 1995;18:501-510).

[21] Lettieri CJ et al., Comparison of adjustable and fixed oral appliances for the treatment of obstructive sleep apnea. *J. Clin. Sleep Med.* 2011; 7:439-445.

[22] Edward T. Chang, Victor Certal, Sungjin A. Song, Soroush Zaghi, Marina Carrasco-Llatas, Carlos Torre, Robson Capasso, Macario Camacho. Dexmedetomidine versus propofol during drug-induced

sleep endoscopy and sedation: a systematic review. *Sleep and Breathing*, 2017, Volume 21, Number 3, Page 727.

[23] Nieuwenhuijs D, Coleman EL, Douglas NJ, et al., (2002) Bispectral index values and spectral edge frequency at different stages of physiologic sleep. *Anesth. Analg.* 94:125–129, table of contents.

[24] Kezirian J, Eric & Hohenhorst, Winfried & de vries, Nico. (2011). Drug-induced sleep endoscopy: The VOTE classification. European archives of oto-rhino-laryngology : official journal of the European Federation of Oto-Rhino-Laryngological Societies (EUFOS): affiliated with the German Society for Oto-Rhino-Laryngology - *Head and Neck Surgery*. 268. 1233-6. 10.1007/s00405-011-1633-8.

[25] Herzog M, Maurer JT. [Drug-induced sedation endoscopy-quo vadis?: Review and outlook]. HNO. 2017 Feb;65(2):125-133. doi: 10.1007/s00106-016-0329-1.

INDEX

A

B

C

I

L

M

N

O

T

U

V

W

Y